Sudden Menopause

DEDICATION

IN DEDICATION TO MY SPECIAL FRIEND, KELLY SALVO
MOREY, WHOSE LIFE WAS A TESTAMENT TO THE
RESILIENCE OF THE HUMAN SPIRIT.

Ordering

Trade bookstores in the U.S. and Canada please contact:

Publishers Group West
1700 Fourth Street, Berkeley CA 94710
Phone: (800) 788-3123   Fax: (510) 528-3444

Hunter House books are available at bulk discounts for textbook course
adoptions; to qualifying community, healthcare, and government organizations;
and for special promotions and fundraising. For details please contact:

Special Sales Department
Hunter House Inc., PO Box 2914, Alameda CA 94501-0914
Phone: (510) 865-5282   Fax: (510) 865-4295
E-mail: ordering@hunterhouse.com

Individuals can order our books from most bookstores,
by calling toll-free: **(800) 266-5592,**
or from our website at **www.hunterhouse.com**

Sudden Menopause

Restoring Health
and Emotional Well-Being

Debbie DeAngelo, R.N.C., B.S.N.

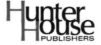

Hunter House Inc., Publishers
PO Box 2914
Alameda CA 94501-0914

Library of Congress Cataloging-in-Publication Data

DeAngelo, Debbie.
Sudden menopause : restoring health and emotional well-being /
Debbie DeAngelo.—1st ed.
p. cm.
Includes bibliographical references and index.
ISBN 0-89793-325-7 (pbk.) — ISBN 0-89793-326-5 (cl.)
1. Menopause—Miscellanea. 2. Menopause—Complications. 3. Women—Health
and hygiene. I. Title.
RG186 .D434 2000
618.1'75—dc21   00-143905

Project Credits

Cover Design: Jinni Fontana
Book Production: Hunter House
Developmental and Copy Editor: Kelley Blewster
Proofreader: David Marion
Indexer: Kathy Talley-Jones
Acquisitions Editor: Jeanne Brondino
Associate Editor: Alexandra Mummery
Editorial and Production Assistant: Emily Tryer
Acquisitions and Marketing Assistant: Lori Covington
Sales and Marketing Assistant: Earlita Chenault
Customer Service Manager: Christina Sverdrup
Order Fulfillment: Joel Irons
Administrator: Theresa Nelson
Computer Support: Peter Eichelberger
Publisher: Kiran S. Rana

Printed and Bound by Publishers Press, Salt Lake City, Utah
Manufactured in the United States of America
9 8 7 6 5 4 3 2 1   First Edition   01 02 03 04 05

Table of Contents

Important Note

The material in this book is intended to provide a review of information regarding sudden menopause. Every effort has been made to provide accurate and dependable information. The contents of this book have been compiled through professional research and in consultation with medical professionals. However, health-care professionals have differing opinions, and advances in medical and scientific research are made very quickly, so some of the information may become outdated.

Therefore, the publisher, authors, and editors, and the professionals quoted in the book cannot be held responsible for any error, omission, or dated material. The authors and publisher assume no responsibility for any outcome of applying the information in this book in a program of self-care or under the care of a licensed practitioner. If you have questions concerning your nutrition or diet, or about the application of the information described in this book, consult a qualified health-care professional.

Foreword

"Fire!" "Terrorist!" "War!"

Certain words in our language elicit immediate, intensely emotional responses. "Cancer!" should be considered one of these types of words.

In *Sudden Menopause,* Debbie DeAngelo, R.N.C., B.S.N., relates her personal experience with cancer—that of ovarian cancer at the age of 26—and how it lead to an unnatural, unexpected, and difficult-to-treat unwellness that she would eventually recognize as the syndrome of "sudden menopause."

A nurse and health educator by profession, she found herself on the "other side" of the health care system. The intensely emotional and medically confusing experience of sudden menopause taught her about this seldomly spoken of, often misunderstood, and sorely untreated medical condition. She sought explanations and understanding and treated herself—comprehensively. This book represents the next step, one typical of any educator worth her salt.

In *Sudden Menopause,* she relates her experience and provides a comprehensive resource that will guide others who suffer from sudden menopause seek control, understanding, restored health, and well-being. It is a guide—long overdue and available nowhere else—to the experience of sudden menopause. It is a "how to" that can help the reader deal with her own struggles and symptoms from the premature cessation of natural female hormones provided by the ovaries. It also provides guidance on how to anticipate and avoid the long-term health problems to which sudden menopause exposes the women who experience it (essential preventative care that should be part of every medical experience in today's proactive, holistic, health-care environment).

From its thorough explanation of what sudden menopause is, to its review of treatments from herbs to hormones, *Sudden Menopause* is designed to provide the reader with the knowledge required to treat her own symptoms. And, as only a nurse educator can do, Debbie DeAngelo provides motivation to regain control, maximize health, and improve quality of life. It is both a great clinical reference and a personal guide to overcoming fear and feeling better.

Sudden Menopause is an outstanding reference for those who need to understand the experience of unexpected or premature menopause because "someone you know" is going through it. It is also an excellent guide for physicians and health-care providers who treat patients with these or similar conditions. As the author notes in her introduction, it bridges the gap between scientific fact (what we know) and anecdotal information (what we think or have experienced). Debbie DeAngelo also includes a thorough bibliography, list of menopause resources, and recommended reading that offer further opportunities to know more and are the best I have read on this subject matter to date.

As a physician specializing in women's health, I have seen many women struggle with the symptoms and emotions of sudden menopause that Debbie DeAngelo had to discover and manage on her own. Some of their stories are related in the author's outstanding use of case studies to illustrate issues and problems that patients face. Through *Sudden Menopause,* we can all learn from their experiences, while we dispell misunderstanding and promote compassion and well-being. It is "one woman's story" offered for the benefit of us all. So, while "Earthquake!" and "Cancer!" might still be words that elicit fear, "Sudden Menopause!" should not.

BRIAN STARK, DO
Clinical Faculty, Primary Care Partners
Hamot Family Practice Residency
Erie, Pennsylvania
April 2001

Preface

I have an 8-inch scar that begins above my navel and travels down the entire length of my abdomen. It is a daily reminder of the two surgeries I underwent 11 years ago to rid myself of ovarian cancer.

I was 26 years old and really having the time of my life. I was basically a newlywed; I had been married only 2 years. My husband and I had just purchased our first house (a fixer-upper), as well as a dog to complete the picture. I was practicing as a registered nurse at a women's center. Much of my time at work was spent performing health counseling, conducting health screenings, teaching classes, and speaking publicly on women's health issues.

One day while at work, I experienced some very heavy bleeding during my menstrual period. It happened only that day, but I was alarmed because such an occurrence was abnormal for me. When I called my doctor's office, I was assured that erratic bleeding was not abnormal in a woman of my age. The doctor's staff told me that it was probably due to stress or an ovarian cyst, and to call back the next day if the problem persisted.

Although the heavy bleeding subsided the same day it started, I scheduled an appointment anyway. Since supposedly I was experiencing a problem that didn't need to be addressed immediately, I had to wait about 4 months for an appointment in my doctor's very busy practice.

As the months passed, I felt perfectly fine. I was able to function 100 percent both at work and at home. However, a few weeks before my appointment, the heavy bleeding returned. Again, it lasted only 1 day. In retrospect I think it might have been a sign from above, just in case I was tempted to cancel my doctor's appointment.

Finally, the day of my doctor's appointment arrived. As I was ushered into the examination room and prepared for the pelvic exam, all of the less-serious reasons why a 26-year-old woman would experience a few episodes of heavy bleeding ran through my mind.

After my doctor entered the room and asked me the standard health questions, she began the pelvic exam. During the exam, we were talking about life in general when she suddenly began concentrating her efforts on my left side.

After deeply palpating my abdomen with a perplexed look on her face, she said, "I feel a mass on your left ovary." I was stunned into silence. Staring blankly at her I finally replied, "Couldn't it be a cyst?" "No," she said, "it's a solid growth. However, given your age and unremarkable family history, I am 99.9 percent sure it is not cancer."

Although my brain heard her words, my heart knew she was wrong. At that very moment an intuitive sense washed over me confirming that it was indeed cancer. I had never felt such a strong "gut instinct" in my life. How could I explain to my doctor what I already knew?

Over the next few weeks I was scheduled for numerous diagnostic tests: ultrasound, CT scan, upper and lower GI series. I did everything in my power to ensure that I received these tests as soon as possible. The tests revealed only that I had a fairly large mass on my left ovary—and one on my right ovary, as well.

Was it cancer? No one knew. The tests ordered to shed more light on the situation did nothing but prove inconclusive. The next step was surgery to remove the tumors.

On 17 May 1990 I was formally diagnosed with ovarian cancer and underwent a hysterectomy with removal of both my ovaries. Over the course of the next 2 months, I had further surgery and treatment for the cancer.

Aside from frequent follow-up exams and tests over the next few years, my treatment was complete. My oncologist pronounced a clean bill of health. I hoped he was right. After 3 months of doctors, tests, and hospitals, it was now time to resume my life.

Although I opted for hormone replacement therapy almost immediately, I found that after about a year I was not my same old self. I went from doctor to doctor trying to effectively manage the night sweats and vaginal dryness. These issues were much easier for my doctors to address than the cognitive problems I developed.

I began noticing changes in my short-term memory and verbal abilities. My doctors were at a loss to explain these. I am certain if I had been 56 instead of 26, they would have told me it was a sign of aging—and I might have believed it. But a previously sharp 26-year-old woman in a mental fog? I didn't think so.

Thus began my search for answers. I refused to accept that I would never feel any better. Maybe my body would never be the same as it was prior to surgery, but I was certain I could return to a comparable state of well-being.

As I researched information related to a sudden menopause (in my case surgically induced), I realized why the doctors were at such a loss to help me. The information I found was diffuse and scanty. There was not a plethora of knowledge, but there was enough to validate what I was feeling.

I then began paying closer attention to the women in my menopause classes and health-counseling sessions. I also extensively interviewed dozens of suddenly menopausal women. Upon questioning these women—most of whom underwent hysterectomy with ovarian removal, had pelvic radiation or some form of chemotherapy, or were diagnosed with an eating disorder that resulted in cessation of periods—many admitted that their menopausal symptoms were not well controlled. They stated that often their doctors and nurses did not address the problems they were having. Some women were unaware that their symptoms were related to sudden menopause.

Sudden menopause is radically different from natural menopause. With natural menopause, the body gradually transitions from higher hormone levels to lower hormone levels. This progression happens over a period of several years, allowing the body to adjust. Many women who undergo a natural menopause will report physical and emotional changes, but for the most part, these changes are either tolerable or easily managed. This is not the case with sudden menopause, which normally comes on fast and furiously. Hormone levels can literally plummet overnight, shocking the body into chaos. Easing menopausal changes in these women requires a greater degree of attention and management.

As my dismay and compassion for women suffering from sudden menopause mounted, I decided I owed it to them and to myself to do something. Over the years, I'd been able to help myself and the many women I'd encountered in my nursing career. It was now time to share my knowledge and experience with a wider audience so they could benefit as well. I asked myself what would have helped me the most when I was struggling. The answer was perfectly clear: a comprehensive resource that provided tips for alleviating my menopausal changes while educating me on how to prevent the long-term health issues for which sudden menopause placed me at risk. This revelation served as the impetus for my writing *Sudden Menopause: Restoring Health and Emotional Well-Being*.

Sudden Menopause is designed to provide you with a way of solving your menopausal woes, while educating and motivating you to achieve optimal health and well-being. The chapter on symptomatic relief provides you with many coping strategies that will help with the most commonly reported menopausal changes.

Although it may be tempting to begin taking vitamins and herbs, first read the chapter on dietary supplements. It will help you to use them safely and responsibly.

The same is true for hormone replacement therapy (HRT). Although many women who experience a sudden menopause find relief through HRT, not every woman is a candidate for this therapy. The information contained in this book will help you to make an informed decision regarding HRT.

The information I have included on osteoporosis and heart disease is crucial, because once you have been through a sudden menopause, your risk for both conditions skyrockets. However, there are many ways you can lower your risk.

The last chapter, titled "Creating Health," helps you to pull together all of the lifestyle information provided in the previous chapters. It also recognizes the important contributions of emotional and spiritual well-being to overall health.

Finally, each chapter offers suggestions for questions to discuss with your doctor.

A special feature of *Sudden Menopause* is the many case histories I've included from women I've worked with. Their stories, which offer perspectives on numerous and varied issues related to sudden menopause, will encourage you that, no matter what the condition that led to your sudden menopause, and no matter what your resulting symptoms, there is hope.

Although every woman's sudden menopause is as unique as the woman herself, and changes do not occur overnight, I am certain of the following:

▨ You can improve the quality of your life.

▨ You can regain control.

▨ You can feel better.

— **Debbie DeAngelo, R.N.C., B.S.N.**

Acknowledgements

I am deeply grateful to the countless women who gave their time and shared their stories of sudden menopause so that other women may benefit.

Thank you to Patti DiPanfilo, whose way with words polished mine. Your contributions were invaluable.

A special thank you to Marci Shimoff, coauthor of *Chicken Soup for the Woman's Soul*, for steering me in the right direction.

I would also like to thank the staff at Hunter House—especially Jeanne Brondino, Alex Mummery, and Kelley Blewster—for their guidance and support.

To my family and friends: your love and support nourish and inspire me. I am especially appreciative of my husband, Mark, who fills my heart with joy, and am indebted to my brother, Chris, who patiently addressed endless pharmaceutical questions.

1

Sudden Menopause:
What Is It?

While having lunch with two of my close friends, I expressed frustration over trying to find information about sudden menopause. They both paused, stared at me blankly, and asked, "What is that?"

I explained that since my ovaries were removed at the time of my hysterectomy, I entered menopause instantaneously, instead of naturally, over a period of years. One of my friends said, "You went through menopause at your age? You're only 26!"

At that moment I realized why I was unable to find much information about sudden menopause. Many people either do not know about the condition or do not understand it.

An Information Gap

Although the level of awareness about natural menopause has increased over the years, the level of awareness about sudden menopause has remained low. This gap in information does not exist only among the general public; health-care professionals also have limited knowledge about what a woman experiences when she is thrown into sudden menopause.

The subject often is glossed over by physicians when they explain the aftereffects of a total hysterectomy or the potential side effects of chemotherapy. Because sudden menopause usually is the result of a hysterectomy with removal of the ovaries, or of a condition that results in ovarian damage, it often takes a backseat to the "pressing" medical problem that caused the sudden menopause. To the physician, the sudden menopause may be looked upon as secondary in importance, but to the woman facing the possibility of an instant change or who is in the throes of severe hot flashes or memory loss, its importance is very real.

Sudden menopause can result from a variety of conditions that instantly render a woman's ovaries incapable of producing the crucial female hormones estrogen and progesterone, as well as the male hormone testosterone. This immediate depletion throws the woman's body into a hormonal tailspin. Sudden menopause can be induced by surgical intervention or by ovarian malfunction or damage. Let's take a look at each of these circumstances.

Surgical Intervention

DORIS is a 40-year-old schoolteacher who began experiencing heavy bleeding during her periods. She also noticed that she was making more frequent trips to the bathroom to urinate. She went to her gynecologist, who performed a pelvic exam and an ultrasound of her reproductive organs. She was told that she had two large uterine fibroid tumors (noncancerous), and that one was pressing on her bladder

Doris's doctor recommended and performed a hysterectomy. Both of her ovaries were removed at the same time because she was told and she believed that she was getting closer to menopause and "did not need them anyway." When I met with her, she was in the throes of sudden menopause. One comment she made remains clearly etched in my mind: "I didn't even know I had options other than a hysterectomy."

The greatest challenge I faced while working with Doris was helping her to work through her feelings of guilt. In retrospect, she realized that she had completely turned her health needs over to her doctor and abandoned any responsibility for her treatment and its outcome. Once I was able to help her focus on the present instead of dwelling in the past, we discovered strategies to help her cope with her anxiety and night sweats. She enrolled in a yoga class so that she could learn relaxation strategies and proper breathing techniques. These helped her deal with the night sweats as well as the anxiety. Dietary modification and changes in her sleeping environment also contributed to reducing the frequency and severity of her night sweats.

———

Hysterectomy is the second most commonly performed surgery in the United States. Approximately 600,000 hysterectomies are performed annually, with the ovaries removed in about half of these cases.[1]

A total or complete hysterectomy is a surgical procedure in which the uterus and cervix are removed. The term oophorectomy (or ovariectomy) refers to the removal of the ovaries, either one (unilateral) or both (bilateral). The fallopian tubes also may be removed in a procedure called salpingectomy. Therefore, when the ovaries and the fallopian tubes are removed along with the uterus, the procedure is called hysterectomy with bilateral salpingo-oophorectomy (BSO).

According to the National Center for Health Statistics, 45.5 percent of all women who undergo a hysterectomy have their ovaries removed at the same time.[2] In some cases, surgery is performed to remove only one ovary; even though the other ovary remains, sudden menopause can occur if the blood flow to the remaining ovary is compromised during surgery.

Commonly cited reasons why hysterectomies are performed include the following:

- **Pelvic inflammatory disease (PID)**—The phrase pelvic inflammatory disease is a generalized term for an infection in the uterus and/or fallopian tubes and ovaries. It is primarily a result of sexually transmitted disease that has spread into the pelvic region. Signs and symptoms of PID may include abdominal pain, mid- to lower back pain, fever, nausea, vomiting, foul-smelling vaginal discharge, pain or bleeding during or after intercourse, and burning upon urination.

- **Endometriosis**—This condition occurs when tissue from the endometrium (the lining of the uterus) attaches itself to other organs, usually in the pelvic area. Organs often affected include the fallopian tubes, ovaries, bladder, and bowel. Since the tissue originated inside of the uterus, it responds to the monthly hormonal cycle in the same way the uterus does. It builds and grows, then breaks down and bleeds. The inflammation and internal bleeding can result in the formation of scar tissue and symptoms such as pelvic pain, painful intercourse, heavy menstrual flow, fatigue, painful bowel movements, constipation, and diarrhea. Endometriosis also is a cause of infertility.

- **Uterine fibroid tumors**—Fibroid tumors, or myomas, are very common and almost always benign (noncancerous). They originate from the muscle tissue of the uterine wall and can grow outward or inward. Small fibroids usually do not create problems, but large ones or clusters of fibroids can cause symptoms, including heavy, prolonged, or irregular menstrual bleeding; abdominal swelling; pelvic or back pain; constipation; and frequent urination.

- **Uterine prolapse**—When the uterus "drops" from its normal position and protrudes through the vagina, it is said to have prolapsed. The normal uterus is anchored in place by ligaments, muscles, and fascia, but over the years, the uterus may change position. It can drop straight down, or tip forward or backward. Childbirth or obesity may entice the uterus to descend. Symptoms of prolapse may include pressure and heaviness in the vaginal region, a feeling of heaviness in the lower abdomen, lower backaches, and urinary frequency and incontinence.

- **Menorrhagia/metrorrhagia**—The term menorrhagia refers to excessive or prolonged menstrual bleeding. Metrorrhagia refers to uterine bleeding between periods. A variety of conditions can result in one or both of these problems. Possible causes include fibroids, polyps, ovarian cysts, hyperplasia, birth control pills, hormonal imbalances, stress, or cancer. Menorrhagia and metrorrhagia need to be carefully evaluated.

- **Breast cancer**—Some forms of breast cancer are estrogen-dependent. This means the hormone estrogen fuels their growth. If this is the case, the ovaries may be removed as part of the cancer treatment. Another breast cancer treatment option is the use of a special medication, such as Tamoxifen, that blocks the estrogen receptors on the cancer cells so they are not responsive to estrogen. Since these medications have become available, oophorectomy is less commonly performed for treatment of breast cancer.

- **Uterine, ovarian, and advanced cervical cancer**—The extent of treatment for these cancers depends upon the type of tumor and how it is staged. Uterine cancer and ovarian cancer normally necessitate a hysterectomy. However, unless cervical cancer is advanced, it usually can be treated more conservatively.

It is important to note that, with the exception of cancer, hysterectomy is not the treatment of choice for the above conditions.

Ovarian Malfunction

"I didn't even know I could go through menopause at my age," remarked 28-year-old *TINA*. Tina is a waitress who struggles with anorexia nervosa. She currently is working with a therapist who specializes in eating disorders, and she is making progress. However, the past decade of starving herself, using diuretics and cathartics, and exercising to excess have taken their toll on her body. She has not had a period in several years.

While she was aware that the cessation of periods, vaginal dryness, hot flashes, and thinking problems were a direct result of the eating disorder, she did not realize that she was menopausal. Tina's sudden menopause was due to ovarian malfunction. Her ovaries simply shut down from malnourishment. As Tina's condition gradually improves, it may be possible for her to regain endocrine function and no longer be menopausal. Only time will tell.

———✦———

Besides being surgically induced, sudden menopause also can occur from conditions that inhibit ovarian function. Ovarian damage can result from the following:

- **Anorexia nervosa**—This is a type of eating disorder that is prevalent in young women. Anorectics have a distorted body image and think they are fat. As a result, they minimize their food intake so that they, in effect, starve themselves. Anorectics become obsessed with weight, food, counting calories, and exercising. Over time, their menstrual cycles cease, a condition called amenorrhea.

- **Chemotherapy**—This generally refers to the medications that are used to treat cancer. A combination of agents often is given. Some of these medications can render the ovaries inactive, causing menstruation to cease.

- **Radiation treatment**—This involves the use of radioactive substances to destroy cancer cells. Radiation can be administered externally or internally to a localized region. Radiation that is directed toward the pelvic region can damage the ovaries and cause the menstrual cycle to stop.

- **Medications**—Certain medications also can cause ovarian shutdown. In fact, some medicines are given for just that purpose. For example, Lupron, which is used to treat endometriosis, works by blocking ovarian function.

In some of these cases, the sudden menopause may be temporary and reversible. In others, it is permanent.

Whether sudden menopause follows surgery or ovarian damage, the body may react to the resulting drastic hormonal changes by manifesting symptoms such as hot flashes, night sweats, vaginal dryness, decreased libido, memory loss, and mood changes. In order to comprehend how a woman's body reacts once the ovaries are removed or damaged, it is important to understand how the female reproductive system normally functions.

The Menstrual Cycle

A common misconception that exists about a woman's monthly cycle is that it begins and ends in the uterus. Although a great deal of activity occurs in this region, the entire process is orchestrated by the brain.

The Brain

Located within the brain is a structure called the hypothalamus. It communicates intimately with the pituitary gland, which sits below it, to regulate the endocrine system. The endocrine system consists of specific glands that secrete hormones to activate bodily functions. Some of these hormonal responsibilities include growth and development, fertility and reproduction, metabolism, fluid and electrolyte balance, and stress response.

The hypothalamus produces a variety of releasing hormones that, in turn, cause the pituitary gland to produce a variety of stimulating hormones. These stimulating hormones go directly to the target organs and initiate action. It is important to keep in mind that, although a single organ may be primarily responsible for specific functions, the endocrine system utilizes a team approach. The hormones all work together.

One example of the endocrine system at work is the functioning of the adrenal glands. After corticotropin-releasing factor (CRF) is secreted from the hypothalamus, it travels to the pituitary gland, which then secretes adrenocorticotropic hormone (ACTH).

The target organs for ACTH are the adrenal glands. These small glands are located on the upper portion of the kidneys and are responsible for the production of many hormones. These hormones include mineralocorticoids, which regulate sodium, potassium, and fluid levels; glucocorticoids, which influence metabolism, response to stress, emotional well-being, and the anti-inflammatory response; androgens, which commonly are referred to as the male hormones (predominantly testosterone) and which govern functions such as libido and the development of armpit and pubic hair; and catecholamines, such as epinephrine and norepinephrine, which function to elicit the "fight or flight" response.

A similar hormonal symphony occurs in the thyroid gland. Once again, the process begins with the hypothalamus, which produces thyrotropin-releasing hormone (TRH). TRH travels to the pituitary gland and causes it to produce thyroid-stimulating hormone (TSH). TSH travels through the bloodstream to the thyroid gland, where thyroid hormones and calcitonin are produced. Thyroid hormones govern metabolism, and calcitonin helps to regulate calcium absorption.

As these examples illustrate, the hypothalamus and the pituitary gland secrete a host of hormones that carry out life-sustaining functions. These hormones coexist in harmony, and a change in one of them can upset the delicate balance within the body.

The ovaries are also under the influence of the pituitary gland. They, too, respond to the directions given to them by the brain.

The Ovaries

Like the thyroid and adrenal glands, the ovaries communicate with the brain. Gonadotropin-releasing hormone (GnRH) is secreted from the hypothalamus and travels to the pituitary gland. The pituitary gland produces follicle-stimulating hormone (FSH) and luteinizing hormone (LH), which prepare the reproductive system for a potential pregnancy (See Figure 1.1). This occurs approximately on a monthly basis.

FSH starts the cyclical process by stimulating the ova (eggs) within the ovaries to grow and to produce estrogen. Estrogen then begins to encourage the cells of the endometrium (uterine lining) to proliferate and thicken, and to create an environment conducive to nourishing a fetus. As the estrogen level peaks, LH springs into

---

Figure 1.1: Hormones of the Menstrual Cycle

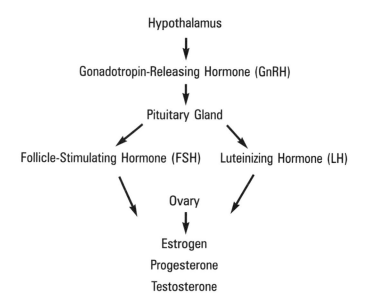

Hypothalamus

↓

Gonadotropin-Releasing Hormone (GnRH)

↓

Pituitary Gland

Follicle-Stimulating Hormone (FSH)   Luteinizing Hormone (LH)

Ovary

↓

Estrogen

Progesterone

Testosterone

---

action and entices one of the eggs to mature and burst forth from the follicle that houses it and to begin its journey through the fallopian tubes to the uterus. This process is called ovulation.

Not only is ovulation necessary for conception to occur, but once ovulation has occurred, the corpus luteum (empty follicle) begins producing progesterone. Progesterone is called the "hormone of pregnancy" and is vital for maintaining a pregnancy. If the ovum does not meet the sperm, the level of progesterone begins to drop off, and the lining of the uterus is shed.

The day menstrual bleeding begins is considered the first day of your period. Based upon a 28-day cycle, days 1 through 14 are called the follicular phase. During that time, only estrogen is produced. Days 15 through 28 make up the luteal phase of the cycle, during which both estrogen and progesterone are present. Small amounts of testosterone are produced by the ovaries throughout the entire menstrual cycle.

Periodically interrupted by pregnancy, the body continues with this rhythmic cycle throughout a woman's life. Menopause, whether gradual or sudden, completes this chapter in a woman's life.

Natural Menopause

When Mother Nature is allowed to progress without interference, menopause generally occurs between the ages of 45 and 55, with an average age of 51. If is occurs before the age of 40, it is termed premature menopause.

Menopause literally means the cessation of menses. It is a woman's last menstrual period. However, it can be viewed only in retrospect, because to be truly menopausal is to be without menstruation for 1 year.

For the vast majority of women, menopause does not occur overnight. Over a period of several years, a woman's body transitions from the fertile years to the nonfertile years. This can begin occurring as many as 10 years before menstruation ceases. This process is referred to as the climacteric.

The term perimenopause often is used to refer to the year or few years preceding menopause, when a woman may begin experiencing erratic periods and changes such as hot flashes, night sweats, and vaginal dryness. Some women do not experience these bothersome changes until menopause actually occurs.

Other changes that may occur over a period of months or years include palpitations, mood changes, dizziness, insomnia, cognitive changes, and urinary frequency. However, every woman is an individual and responds to the gradually decreasing and imbalanced hormone levels in her own unique way. Some women will experience a few of these changes, some will experience many of these changes, and some will experience none at all.

Approximately 2 to 4 years before the last period, ovulation becomes irregular and eventually ceases. The ovaries continue to produce some estrogen, but progesterone production is dependent on ovulation. Therefore, estrogen builds up the lining of the uterus, but if ovulation does not occur, progesterone is not present to cause the uterine lining to slough off on a regular basis. Instead, a woman bleeds erratically as the endometrium breaks away uncleanly, due to the months of buildup. This can lead to irregular cycles—light flow, heavy flow, skipped periods, or more or less frequent periods.

When menopause does occur, it is marked by the cessation of menses. Other changes that occur include the completion of the fertile years, a decline in levels of estrogen and testosterone, and the termination of progesterone production from the ovaries.

What does the brain think about all this? It begins a flurry of activity in response to the declining levels of estrogen and progesterone. In an attempt to compensate for the low levels of hormones, the pituitary gland puts out high amounts of FSH and LH. During perimenopause, periodic bursts of activity from the ovaries may temporarily increase the amount of estrogen. If occasional ovulation is still occurring, small amounts of progesterone also may be produced, and pregnancy can occur. However, over time, the ovaries cannot be stimulated, and the levels of estrogen and progesterone continue to decrease, despite the high levels of FSH and LH. An FSH blood test can be performed to gauge the activity in the ovaries and the response of the pituitary gland. If the FSH level is consistently over 40 mIU/ml (40 thousandths of International Units per milliliter), menopause has occurred.[3]

It is important to note that although the ovaries are not producing as much estrogen and testosterone as they did prior to menopause, they still are manufacturing small amounts of the hormones. In addition, the adrenal glands and fat tissue convert hormones into estrogen and produce testosterone. These hormonal fluctuations are responsible for the changes that occur in a woman's body during perimenopause and postmenopause.

The symptoms of menopause, as well as their timing and duration, are just as individual as the menstrual cycle itself. Women can find as many similarities in their experiences as they can find nuances specific to themselves. One of those shared experiences is that natural menopause is a gradual process. The body has years to adjust to it. This is important, because the transitioning process—with the integrity of the ovaries remaining intact and producing hormones—marks the great difference between a natural menopause and a sudden menopause.

Chapter Highlights

- Sudden menopause most commonly results from a hysterectomy with removal of the ovaries. Under this circumstance, it is permanent and irreversible.

- Ovarian malfunction secondary to anorexia nervosa, some forms of chemotherapy, pelvic radiation, and certain medications targeted at suppressing ovarian function can result in sudden menopause. Sometimes sudden menopause due to ovarian malfunction is temporary and reversible.

- Ovarian hormones work synergistically and interdependently with all of the other hormones in the body. Sometimes an imbalance in one area can trigger hormone discord in another area.

Doc Talk

- Ask your doctor to explain how and why your body was thrown into a sudden menopause.

- Discuss how your body may compensate for the sudden reduction in ovarian hormones.

- Talk to your doctor about what you might feel like during your sudden menopause. Together with her or him formulate a health plan to deal with these changes.

2

"What's Going On Now?": Menopausal Changes

As I sat in the hospital bed the day after my hysterectomy (with my ovaries removed), my doctor asked me, "Are you having hot flashes yet?" Over the next few days, I was asked that question repeatedly. In fact, I became hypervigilant about awaiting the arrival of hot flashes. "Where are they? Why aren't I having them yet? Am I normal?" I soon realized that no two people respond to the same circumstances in the exact same way. Although most women do experience immediate hot flashes after the removal of their ovaries, I did not.

One month after surgery, I began estrogen replacement therapy (ERT). During the next year and a half, I felt no different from how I'd felt prior to surgery. I experienced very few hot flashes or other symptoms. Shortly thereafter, however, I began noticing some subtle changes indicative of hormone deficiency. I called my doctor and asked her to increase my dosage of estrogen.

Over the next several months, I failed to notice much improvement. I continued to experience vaginal dryness, as well as some changes in my memory and my level of concentration. I tried herbal preparations and various vitamins. Although these remedies work for many women, I did not experience a noticeable difference. The vaginal dryness progressively worsened and was accompanied by a significant decrease in libido. During this time, I had my estrogen levels checked twice, and the results were "normal."

In near desperation, I approached my family doctor for help. He was very sympathetic, but could only offer two suggestions. The first was to expedite the appointment I had with my gynecologist. The second suggestion was to undergo psychological counseling to determine if I was experiencing an adjustment problem. Since I knew I was not crazy, I chose the first option.

As I waited for my scheduled gynecology appointment, I became fed up. I didn't care what the tests showed. My body was screaming with symptoms characteristic of hormone deficiency. I set to work researching my problems, and then went to my gynecologist equipped with information and determination.

My doctor agreed to try adding testosterone to my estrogen therapy. I also suggested performing a maturation test on the cells of my vaginal walls. The vaginal cells are very sensitive to changes in estrogen levels. The maturation index, commonly performed during a Pap test, can confirm low estrogen levels. More accurate information is gleaned by performing the maturation test at regular intervals. Not surprising to me, the tests showed an estrogen deficiency. This was confirmation that I understood what was happening to my body. We experimented with an estrogen that was chemically identical to what my body produced, as well as adding testosterone to my regimen. Not only was it a relief to find out I was reading my body correctly, but I also began to feel pretty good once the medication changes were made.

What is the moral of this story? It is that persistence pays off. According to a study commissioned by the North American Menopause Society, most women seek outside sources of menopause information in addition to that provided by their doctors. In fact, of the 750 women surveyed, the majority noted that they turned to reading materials, friends, family members, and the media for guidance.[1] For those undergoing sudden menopause in particular, seeking outside information may prove even more important in the quest for a return to feeling good, since data readily available to medical professionals about this phenomenon is still limited. As indicated by my own difficulty finding useful information following my hysterectomy, sudden menopause simply isn't yet granted the same status in medical journals and self-help literature that natural menopause receives. For that reason, some digging may be necessary—and doing so may make the difference in how satisfied you are with the health-care plan you work out with your physician.

As long as accurate information is obtained, outside sources can introduce you to ideas and suggestions to which you would not otherwise have been exposed. Access to information can give you a clearer vision about the approach you would like to take toward your specific experiences. Sharing what you learn with your physician will help her to fine-tune her suggestions to meet your needs, will foster a partnership between the two of you, and will enable her to use the knowledge to help other women.

A Wave of Changes

Symptoms that can occur after a sudden menopause—as well as their onset and duration—vary from woman to woman. Although the symptoms for sudden menopause and natural menopause are generally the same, they are immediate and often more severe for women with sudden menopause. Commonly reported changes include the following:

hot flashes
night sweats
loss of libido
vaginal dryness and infections
urinary incontinence
bladder infections
difficulty concentrating
decreased attention span
memory deficits
mood swings
anxiety
irritability
depression

fatigue

joint pain

dry skin

sleep disturbances

palpitations

weight changes

headaches

Note: Osteoporosis and heart disease also are long-term concerns.

Keep in mind that while you may experience some of these changes, it is unlikely that you will experience all of them.

Measures that may result in some relief also will vary from woman to woman. Often, it takes a process of trial and error to find the key to restoring balance in a woman's life. This can be a tedious process, especially if you are not a candidate for HRT or if you do not want to use hormones.

In a society that is accustomed to quick fixes, it is easy to get frustrated trying to find the therapies that will work best for you. It does not help matters that your life continues at its usual frenetic pace, while at the same time you are trying to cope with these additional concerns. This tends to increase your stress level because you are not functioning at 100 percent. And if this situation is accompanied by an actual or perceived lack of support from family, friends, colleagues, or health professionals, loneliness and despair may soon follow. Additionally, natural menopause happens over time, making it easier to adjust to the changes. With sudden menopause, a woman doesn't have this luxury. She is bombarded with the changes immediately.

It is important to remember, however, that steps can be taken to alleviate symptoms, or at least to make them tolerable. HRT can provide very effective relief, but it is not the only option. HRT will be discussed in greater detail later in the book. Here I would like to focus on some of the changes that are most commonly reported during sudden menopause. I'll also discuss some coping strategies for each symptom and include some stories from women who have lived through them.

Hot Flashes: Smoldering Ember or Towering Inferno?

PEG, a 33-year-old aerobics instructor, entered into sudden menopause while battling an eating disorder. She stated, "I was having numerous hot flashes daily and at night. The bed sheets were soaked. Some doctors told me to live with it. That's a terrible way to tell someone to live."

Peg wasn't aware that she was in menopause as a consequence of her eating disorder. Once we identified the source of her symptoms, we began looking at her options, and she decided on hormone replacement therapy.

———

Perhaps the most notorious of all menopausal symptoms is the hot flash, or as I like to call it, the power surge. The hot flash is notorious because it is a somewhat universal experience, one that women can discuss and compare. Various sources note that hot flashes affect as many as 75 percent to 90 percent of all menopausal women in the United States.

In her book *Estrogen,* Dr. Lila Nachtigall states that 50 percent of women who experience hot flashes will stop having them within a year. For 30 percent of women, hot flashes will last up to 2½ years, and the remaining 20 percent will experience them for many years. A very small number, 2 percent to 3 percent, will experience hot flashes throughout the rest of their lives.[2]

It has been suggested that hot flashes occur because of the changing levels of hormones—decreased estrogen and increased FSH and LH—as well as the increased activity of the neurotransmitter norepinephrine. These fluctuating levels affect the body's temperature-regulating system in the hypothalamus. Consequently, the blood vessels dilate and constrict irregularly, which results in a warm, flushed feeling followed by a cool, clammy feeling.

Many women can sense a hot flash coming on before it actually occurs. A hot flash can range from a feeling of mild warmth to one of intense heat. The feeling can be limited to the upper body, face, and neck, or it can be felt throughout the entire body.

Hot flashes can be accompanied by a flushed appearance to the skin, sweating, dizziness, and heart palpitations. The duration and frequency of hot flashes also vary. Reportedly, the average length of a hot flash is four minutes; however, some women report having hot flashes that last up to an hour. Hot flashes can occur occasionally or as frequently as one right after another all day long.

Every woman's pattern of hot flashes is different. For example, I do not have episodic heat waves during the day, but my body temperature is elevated during the night. I describe it as feeling like my engine is idling fast all night long. Suzanne, a 46-year-old secretary, experienced a sudden menopause due to chemotherapy for breast cancer. She described her hot flashes by saying, "I felt like standing up and ripping off all of my clothes."

If you are troubled by hot flashes or night sweats, the following suggestions may help you find relief.

Coping Strategies

Keep a hot-flash diary.

Hot flashes may be triggered by a variety of situations or substances. By keeping track of the frequency, duration, and severity of your hot flashes—as well as the precipitating factors, such as the foods you ate beforehand or the herbal supplements that seem to help—you may see a pattern emerge. This will help you to better manage your episodes by, for example, eliminating foods that tend to cause them.

There's no need to feel embarrassed.

Unless you exhibit extreme sweating and facial redness or begin tearing at your clothes, hot flashes are seldom noticeable to others. Also, some studies have linked hot flashes to stress. If you continue to worry about them, you may find that you experience them more often.

Try to control the room temperature.

Keep the temperature in the room slightly cool. Ventilate the environment at work and at home with a small fan. This is especially helpful at night if you are prone to night sweats. Utilize air conditioning, if available, and avoid enclosed areas.

Try to adjust your body temperature.

Dress in layers so that you can shed your outer garments when a hot flash comes on. Wear natural fibers such as cotton, as many synthetics don't breathe easily, which can trigger hot flashes.

If excessive sweating is a problem, however, avoid wearing garments made from cotton immediately next to your skin, as cotton will simply absorb the perspiration and leave the garment wet. There's nothing worse than being stuck for several hours with a cold, damp T-shirt clinging to your flesh! As an alternative, try garments made of the new "moisture management" fabrics, originally designed for sports. These are synthetic fabrics, but they breathe, and they also "wick" the perspiration away from your skin to the outside of the garment, where it can evaporate. Reputable sports and outdoor retailers are good sources for casual clothes and activewear that will leave you feeling dry after a bout of sweating.

Avoid shirts with high necklines, as they may feel stifling during a hot flash. Take a cool shower or go swimming. Avoid hot tubs and saunas, as well as sunbathing. Drink cool liquids, and exercise in air conditioning. Avoid hot liquids, spicy foods, sugar, caffeine, alcohol, and smoking.

At night, wear lightweight pajamas. Keep a glass of cool water at your bedside, along with a bowl of cool water and a washcloth to sponge yourself. Avoid flannel sheets and electric blankets. Also, many women swear that sticking your feet outside of the covers helps to cool down the body temperature immediately. (Try this; it actually works!)

Practice stress-management techniques.

Regularly practicing some of the following techniques can help to lessen the effects of a hot flash, as well as to prevent their occurrence:

deep breathing

progressive relaxation

guided imagery/visualization

meditation

yoga

therapeutic massage

listening to soothing music or relaxation tapes

learning time-management skills

communicating assertively

Exercise.

Exercise improves your circulation and helps your body to work more efficiently. This includes the endocrine system. Exercise also helps to manage stress, which influences hot flashes.

Sweating is your body's way of cooling down, and it is necessary when exercising. However, to prevent overheating, it helps to exercise during the coolest part of the day and to perform indoor activities in a well-ventilated or air-conditioned area.

Change your diet.

Try incorporating soy products or ground flaxseed into your diet. Various studies have shown them to be effective in reducing the frequency and lessening the severity of hot flashes and night sweats.

Try supplements.

Learn how vitamins, minerals, and herbs work. Also learn about their potential side effects and contraindications. Then you can experiment with nutritional supplements to find the ones that benefit you most. I will discuss supplements in more detail in Chapter 5, but here are a few common ones to consider for relief from hot flashes:

vitamin E

oil of evening primrose (or other essential fatty acids)

vitamin B complex

vitamin C

calcium

ginseng*

vitex**

dong quai

black cohosh*

anise*

fennel*

fenugreek*

red clover*

red raspberry

spearmint

* contains phytoestrogens, which produce estrogen-like effects

** contains phytoprogesterone, which produces progesterone-like effects.

Consider medication.

By far, one of the most frequently cited reasons for beginning estrogen replacement therapy is to help with hot flashes. Estrogen is very effective in eliminating them or at least decreasing their frequency and severity. For women who should avoid estrogen, progesterone alone can be beneficial (see Chapter 6).

Depending on the reason for your sudden menopause, you may not be a candidate for hormones. If some of the previously suggested options have not worked and hormones are not recommended for you, a few medication alternatives exist that you can discuss with your doctor.

Clonidine (Catapres) normally is prescribed for hypertension (high blood pressure), but sometimes it provides relief from hot flashes. Side effects of this medicine may include decreased blood pressure (less likely with the clonidine patch), dizziness, dry mouth, fatigue, nausea, and irritability. Propranolol (Inderal) is prescribed for high blood pressure and chest pain; it may reduce hot flashes as well. Side effects can include fatigue, decreased blood pressure, and nausea.

Currently, a few low-dose antidepressants are being used to control hot flashes. Venlafaxine (Effexor) was recently studied and found to significantly reduce the frequency of hot flashes in breast cancer survivors. Commonly reported side effects included dry mouth, decreased appetite, nausea, and constipation.

"This Is So Embarrassing!": Vaginal and Urinary Tract Symptoms

A 34-year-old saleswoman named MEGAN scheduled a health-counseling session with me after dealing with her menopausal changes for 1 year. A couple of years earlier, she had been diagnosed with endometriosis. Unfortunately, her doctor did not offer her many treatment options. After a year of unsuccessful oral-contraceptive therapy, she opted for a hysterectomy with BSO (see Chapter 1).

Since endometriosis is estrogen-dependent, Megan was not initially placed on hormone replacement therapy. She was able to control some of her menopausal changes using lifestyle and dietary modifications as well as supplements. However, she was looking for more relief. Upon my questioning her about vaginal dryness, she stated, "Yes, I do have that. I had no idea that vaginal dryness was due to low estrogen."

In an attempt to eradicate her hot flashes and moodiness, she was taking just about every vitamin imaginable. The first thing we did was limit her supplements to antioxidants and B complex. We also examined her diet. Although she was eating a diet low in fat, it was also deficient in protein. Adequate protein intake is essential for mental clarity and peace of mind. Megan found moderate relief of her symptoms from these changes, but still required something more to further help with the hot flashes. She didn't care for the taste of soy products, so she began using flaxseed and found it to be very helpful. Even though her doctor did not want to place her on HRT immediately, she was still eligible for an estrogen-based vaginal cream to treat the vaginal dryness. Since she experienced great relief from these strategies, she opted not to go on HRT for the time being.

———

Unlike hot flashes, women tend not to discuss vaginal dryness, decreased libido, vaginal infections, or stress incontinence. However, once the subject is brought up, the floodgates open and questions pour forth. One striking commonality exists among many of the women I counsel: they do not realize that these symptoms are related to a deficiency in ovarian hormones.

During natural menopause, the ovaries continue to produce small amounts of estrogen. By contrast, a woman with sudden menopause, whose ovaries are damaged or removed, is unable to produce estrogen from the ovaries. (Small amounts of estrogen and testosterone continue to be produced from the adrenal glands, the fatty tissue, and the conversion of other hormones by the liver.) Low hormone levels affect women differently. Even though genital and urinary symptoms tend to be the last symptoms to arrive in any menopausal woman, they arrive sooner and more abruptly in a sudden menopausal woman.

One of the possible effects of low hormone levels is a significant impact on the integrity of the vagina. With less estrogen to keep it full and supple, the vagina loses elasticity and lubrication. Blood flow to the genitals also is decreased. The outer layer of cornified (protective) cells, which shields the vagina from irritation and injury, thins out, leaving the vagina tender and vulnerable to infection.

Over the years, the vagina can become shorter and narrower. Diminishing hormone levels also decrease the flow of the vaginal and cervical secretions necessary for lubrication. If the cervix is removed during a hysterectomy, this problem is compounded. Sex can become painful and much less desirable. Desire also may be hampered by decreased levels of estrogen and testosterone.

All of these changes may lead to vaginitis (vaginal infections), vaginal dryness, genital itching and soreness, and a decreased sex drive. Another condition, called atrophic vaginitis, also may develop. This condition is a chronic inflammation of the vagina and is due to an estrogen deficiency rather than to an infection.

Keep in mind that vaginal and vulvar itching, burning, and redness don't always signify an infection or estrogen deficiency. Sometimes these signs and symptoms are caused by an allergic reaction or sensitivity (dermatitis). Substances that trigger dermatitis vary among women, but the condition is usually the result of an irritating product or ingredient coming into contact with the vagina or vulva. Common irritants include fragrances, scented sanitary products, soaps, bubble baths, douches, and spermicides. Further complicating the matter is that some women run a reaction to specific ingredients in lubricants and vaginal yeast infection medicines. Reported culprits include propylene glycol, methylparaben, and butylated hydroxyanisol (BHA). Therefore, it is crucial that a culture is obtained to diagnose a vaginal infection before treatment begins. If symptoms persist despite the fact that no infection is present or after an infection is diagnosed and treated, irritant dermatitis should be suspected. Treatment includes identifying and eliminating the offensive substance and restoring vaginal integrity. Often petrolatum or solid vegetable oil is prescribed.

Estrogen, as we have seen, plays a key role in the proper functioning of the reproductive canal, but it also influences the urinary tract. The tissue that forms the urinary tract is very similar to that of the vagina. As estrogen levels decrease, the urethra becomes thinner and less pliable. It, too, is now more vulnerable to irritation and infection (called urinary tract infections, or UTIs). Other discomforts might include dysuria (painful urination), nocturia (urination at night), and frequency and urgency of urination.

Urinary tract infections were MARIE'S chief complaint. Although prior to menopause she suffered only the occasional UTI, post-menopausally she was bombarded with them. They were accompanied by vaginal dryness.

Marie had her uterus and one ovary removed at the age of 40, but she was unsure of the actual reason. She just said that her doctor recommended the surgery, so she had it. The remaining ovary produced enough hormones so that she did not notice a difference in her overall well-being. However, 7 years later the remaining ovary became polycystic (grew multiple cysts), so she had it removed.

When she came to see me 5 years after this second surgery, Marie, now age 52, reported that the estrogen she was using took care of her menopausal symptoms. What she didn't realize was that the UTIs and the vaginal dryness also were attributed to an estrogen deficiency. Within six weeks of using an estrogen-based vaginal cream and adhering to the suggestions below, she reported dramatic relief.

———————

Some women also may have to deal with urinary stress incontinence. This occurs when a small quantity of urine is excreted when pressure is exerted on the bladder, for example, while exercising, coughing, laughing, sneezing, or lifting.

Addressing genital and urinary tract symptoms is just as important as addressing hot flashes or osteoporosis. The goals of treatment should include experiencing comfortable sex, regaining urinary control, and decreasing or eliminating vaginal and urinary tract infections.

Coping Strategies

Be honest with yourself and your partner.
The first step in dealing with vaginal dryness is admitting to yourself that it is a problem for you. It is just as important that you share this information with your sexual partner, especially since many women begin to avoid sex as it becomes more painful or as their sex drive diminishes. Your partner may interpret this as rejection.

Also, examine your feelings and thoughts about your body. Women who have had a hysterectomy or a mastectomy often undergo drastic changes in body image and self-esteem, which may keep them from engaging in a sexual relationship. If you are having trouble working through these issues, seek professional help and share your feelings with your partner.

Experiment with lubricants.

Using a water-soluble lubricant—such as K-Y Jelly, Surgi-lube, Gyne-moistren, or Astroglide—prior to sex can help you to deal with the discomfort resulting from vaginal dryness. Although this does not replenish the protective layer of vaginal cells, it decreases the threat of injury during intercourse by reducing friction. It also helps you to relax during sex, because you are not as focused on your inability to become fully lubricated. Using petroleum jelly or oils is not recommended, because they are not readily excreted and can become a breeding ground for infection. They also can break down the latex of which most condoms are made. If you suffer from irritant dermatitis, check the ingredient lists on the labels of any lubricants and moisturizing gels you use. Avoid products that contain substances to which you are sensitive.

Try using a moisturizing gel.

Moisturizing gels, such as Replens, represent an alternative to lubricants. Like lubricants, they do not rebuild the protective layer of vaginal cells, but they seem to moisten the cells. They may even delay the loss of the tough outer vaginal lining. Replens is used two to three times per week instead of immediately before sex.

Engage in regular sex.

Regular intercourse keeps the vagina more supple and lubricated by stimulating vaginal secretions and maintaining muscle tone. It also helps to stimulate your sex drive. For the same reasons, increasing foreplay is beneficial. You also may find it more comfortable to take the "top" position during intercourse. Doing so enables you to control the rate and depth of penetration.

If you do not have a partner, masturbation and the use of sexual aids can provide you with the same benefits. If diminished sex drive continues to be a problem, experimenting with the herb damiana or using hormone replacement therapy with testosterone may help.

Perform Kegel exercises.

Kegel exercises strengthen the muscles of the pelvic floor. This helps to increase vaginal tone and support the urinary structures, which in turn improves urinary stress incontinence and heightens sexual pleasure. The hardest part about performing Kegel exercises is identifying the correct muscles to use. The next time you are urinating, try to stop or at least slow down your urine stream. The muscles that you use to do this, the pelvic floor muscles, are the ones that you will strengthen with this exercise. (Do not perform this exercise while urinating.)

To perform the Kegels, contract your pelvic floor muscles for a count of five to 10, release for a count of 10, and repeat. A variation of the exercise is to contract the muscles quickly. To get optimal results, you need to perform at least 100 repetitions of this exercise each day.

It is very easy to fit Kegel exercises into your daily routine, because no one can tell that you are doing them. Perform your repetitions whenever you are standing in a line, sitting at a red light, or watching television. You will not even work up a sweat!

Vaginal cones are available to assist with this exercise. A set consists of cones of various weights that are inserted into the vagina like a tampon and held there to strengthen the muscles. You hold the weights in place by using the muscles of the pelvic floor. You gradually increase the length of time performing the exercise to 15 minutes twice a day. Although the cones are available in stores, professional guidance from your doctor is necessary for proper fit and instructions for use. That is why I recommend working closely with your doctor.

Prevent vaginal infections.

Take measures to prevent vaginal infections and irritation by following these suggestions:

- Do not share underwear, panty hose, bathing suits, or towels. Infectious organisms can be transmitted via shared clothing.

- Wear underwear with a crotch made from cotton instead of nylon or other synthetics, to allow air to circulate and moisture to evaporate. Alternatively, look for underwear made from the same new "wicking" fabrics recommended earlier in this chapter. Reputable athleticwear manufacturers offer these specialty garments. Avoid wearing pajama bottoms to bed, and decrease the length of time that you wear tight-fitting pants or exercise clothing. These garments trap moisture and do not allow air to circulate.

- Do not sit around in a wet bathing suit, and dry your genital area thoroughly after bathing, showering, or swimming. Bacteria and yeast thrive in a warm, moist, dark environment.

- Avoid using bubble bath, bath oils, feminine hygiene sprays, and powders. Also, be aware that detergents and soaps can cause irritation. Don't use any products on your genitals if you have developed a reaction to them in the past. Choose showers over baths.

- Avoid public hot tubs. The chlorine evaporates because of the high temperatures, and disease transmission is possible.

- Refrain from routine douching. It can alter the delicate balance of helpful organisms in the body. Consult your doctor about the recommended frequency and type of douche to use when you feel the need.

- After a bowel movement, pat (rather than wipe) from front to back. This will prevent the introduction of bacteria into the vagina.

- Choose your sexual partners carefully, and use condoms. Infections can be asymptomatic and passed back and forth between partners.

- Take antibiotics only when necessary. If you are prone to vaginal infections, discuss this with your doctor before an antibiotic is prescribed.

- Eat a diet that is low in sugar. A high-sugar diet may encourage yeast infections.

- Try eating cultured yogurt several times a week, if not daily. "Cultured" means that it contains active *Lactobacillus acidophilus*. Not all yogurt has this, so check the label.

Prevent urinary tract infections.

Consider the following tips for preventing urinary tract infections:

- Wear underwear with a crotch made from cotton instead of nylon or other synthetics, to allow air to circulate and moisture to evaporate. Alternatively, look for underwear made from the same new "wicking" fabrics recommended earlier in this chapter. Reputable athleticwear manufacturers offer these specialty garments. Avoid wearing pajama bottoms to bed, and decrease the length of time that you wear tight-fitting pants or exercise clothing. These garments trap moisture and do not allow air to circulate.

- Avoid using bubble bath, bath oils, feminine hygiene sprays, and powders. Also, be aware that detergents and soaps can cause urethral irritation. Choose showers over baths. Don't use any products on your genitals if you have developed a reaction to them in the past.

- Do not hold your urine. Urinate at least every 3 to 4 hours, or more often if you need to. If you have lost some bladder sensation, put yourself on a bladder-training schedule to ensure regular urination. Empty your bladder completely. If you are not sure whether you have emptied it completely, lean forward so that your abdomen rests on your thighs. This pressure over your bladder will push out any remaining urine in your bladder.

- After a bowel movement, pat (rather than wipe) from front to back. This will prevent the introduction of bacteria into the urinary tract.

- Monitor your fluid intake. Drink at least eight glasses of water per day. A minimum of half of your fluid intake should be water. Not only does water help to flush out your bladder, but it also decreases the concentration of your urine, which, left undiluted, can provide a breeding ground for infection. Avoid caffeine, alcohol, and carbonated soda, all of which dehydrate your system.

- Drink one to two glasses of cranberry juice per day. Recent studies on the efficacy of drinking cranberry juice suggest that it is helpful because it contains substances that prevent bacteria from adhering to the walls of the urinary tract. Most commercial cranberry juice has a high sugar content but low juice content, so be sure to read the label carefully. You may want to choose unsweetened cranberry-juice concentrate diluted with water. This may only be available at a health food store. Note: if you suffer from interstitial cystitis, cranberry juice may aggravate the condition.

- Pay attention to your diet. Note which foods bring on symptoms or aggravate them. Research regarding diet and cystitis (bladder infection) is conflicting. Some experts recommend a high-acid diet, and others favor a low-acid diet. If the following suggestions help, then continue with them. Avoid chocolate and spicy foods, because they may irritate the bladder. Decrease your intake of sugar, white flour, fats, and meats to help maintain the acid balance of your urine. Eat cultured yogurt several times a week, if not daily. Besides possibly aggravating UTIs, caffeine, alcohol, acidic fruit juice, tomatoes, spicy foods, and sugar also may aggravate stress incontinence.

⚅ Take measures to prevent constipation. The pressure of a full rectum may prevent the bladder from emptying completely.

⚅ Avoid smoking. Nicotine irritates the bladder and increases the risk of cancer, and smokers cough more, which aggravates stress incontinence.

⚅ Urinate before and after sex. Since sex frequently is a cause of UTIs, if you are sexually active, taking measures to decrease infections is a wise move. Try to drink a glass of water before intercourse to ensure urination afterward. Other helpful hints include minimizing clitoral stimulation, which can irritate the urethra and introduce bacteria; avoiding other activities, such as oral sex, that can introduce bacteria into the urethra; and showering after sex.

Talk with your doctor about available treatments for urinary stress incontinence.

Mild incontinence may be helped simply by incorporating Kegel exercises into your daily routine. More serious cases may require additional treatment, such as medication that helps to constrict the bladder outlet.

Another treatment is the use of a pessary, which is a rubber ring that fits into the vagina—much like a diaphragm—to support the cervix and raise the neck of the bladder. It is commonly used for vaginal prolapse. A fairly new treatment similar to a pessary is a bladder-neck support prosthesis.

A periurethral injection, another treatment option, inserts collagen or your own body fat into the tissue surrounding the urethra to add bulk so that it will close more tightly. There also is a surgical treatment to correct the position of the bladder neck by using sutures or by creating a "sling" from muscle tissue or a prosthetic material.

Experiment with supplements for vaginal and urinary tract health.

Many nutritional supplements exist that can contribute to vaginal and urinary tract health. Below is a brief list of them. Take the time to learn how they work. Also learn their potential side effects and contraindications. Supplements are discussed in greater detail in Chapter 5.

Vaginal symptoms	*Urinary tract symptoms*
vitamin E	cranberry
vitamin B complex	uva ursi
cinnamon	vitamin C
barberry	vitamin A
damiana	vitamin B complex
garlic	magnesium
chamomile	zinc
dandelion	cinnamon
echinacea	dill
goldenseal	garlic

Note: the same herbs listed for hot flashes, the phytohormones, also may relieve vaginal and urinary tract symptoms.

Consider medication.

Many of the changes that lead to vaginal and urinary tract disorders are caused and/or aggravated by a deficiency of ovarian hormones. For that reason, hormones may be prescribed to correct these problems (see Chapter 6).

Most women have endured some type of vaginal infection during their lives. It is extremely important to know which organism caused the infection before the appropriate treatment can begin. If it is a bacterial infection, antibiotics can be prescribed. If you are prone to yeast infections, share this information with your doctor before she prescribes antibiotics, because antibiotics can precipitate a yeast infection.

Treatment for yeast infections is now available over the counter. Gyne-Lotrimin and Monistat are examples of antifungal medications that formerly required a prescription. These medications are effective only for yeast infections, so you must be certain you have a yeast infection. If you suspect that yeast is the culprit but you have never been diagnosed with an infection, call your doctor. Dermatitis of the vagina or vulva that occurs without an accompanying yeast or bacterial infection won't be helped by antibiotics or antifungal medicine. This problem should be treated as a dermatological condition.

Cystitis (bladder infection) requires treatment with antibiotics. If the problem seems related to intercourse, your doctor may prescribe an antibiotic to be taken just before or after sex. If you suffer from recurrent cystitis, your physician may place you on preventive therapy, which consists of taking the antibiotic every day. Another alternative is to receive a prescription with several refills, so that at the first sign of infection you can begin taking the medication.

"Am I Losing My Mind?"

One of the severest cases of sudden menopause I have ever encountered was Olivia's. *OLIVIA* was a 32-year-old bookkeeper for a family-run business who had experienced monthly episodes of significant menstrual pain from endometriosis. Since she had difficulty tolerating oral contraceptives, she underwent numerous laser ablation (removal) procedures over the years to remove the endometrial tissue, which had adhered to her uterus, ovaries, and bowel. However, each surgery just triggered more and more scar tissue, which resulted in more pain.

At the end of her rope, Olivia told her doctor to "take it all out." Immediately after the hysterectomy with BSO, Olivia reported "horrible hourly hot flashes" and "night sweats that keep me up at night." As bad as these were, the problems that she found the most troubling were the memory changes. She sat in my office and cried, "Am I going crazy? Have I lost my mind?"

Over the course of 6 months, Olivia was eventually able to restore the physical and emotional balance in her life. For her, this required a combination of hormone replacement therapy (it took several months of experimenting with low dosages to hit upon a good recipe for her), nutritional changes, soy products, and vitamins.

Not all menopausal women report changes in emotion or in mental functioning (cognition), but those who do find the changes frightening. In fact, many women experiencing memory deficits fear they have early-onset Alzheimer's disease. These changes seem to be more disruptive and unsettling than hot flashes or other physically manifested problems. They can be compounded for the sudden menopausal woman because, as with all the other symptoms, she is experiencing them more immediately than the woman undergoing natural menopause. In addition, she also is dealing with the medical condition that resulted in the sudden menopause. This extra stress can further aggravate the cognitive and emotional problems she is facing.

Frequently cited concerns include irritability, mood swings, anxiety, depression, forgetfulness, difficulty concentrating, decreased attention span, and memory deficits. Compounding the frustration felt over these symptoms is the fact that some physicians do not consider them to be serious or related to menopause. Comments such as "That is not a part of menopause"; "It is stress-related"; "I have never read anything about that"; and "You are just a little depressed right now" still prevail.

This dismissive attitude is demeaning and belittles the hardships with which these women struggle. Women begin to think they are "crazy," especially when an expert fails to validate their experiences. Health-care professionals agree that menopause is an individualized process; it is not the same for everyone. Yet when a woman's symptoms deviate from what is considered normal or typical, it often is assumed that the problems must be "in her head."

Just as the causes of night sweats, palpitations, and urogenital symptoms can be independent of menopause, so can emotional and cognitive changes. They can be indicative of a multitude of illnesses, as well as of stress. For that reason, careful evaluation of these symptoms is necessary to determine their cause. However, in an otherwise healthy, well-adjusted woman who undergoes sudden menopause and then develops emotional changes or begins to feel like she is in a "mental fog" (or a "brain fade," as I like to call it), hormonal insufficiency as a source should be a top consideration.

Although there is a relative shortage of research devoted to exploring the emotional and cognitive changes experienced by surgically menopausal women, studies do exist that suggest a link between these symptoms and hormonal deficiency. For example, a research study conducted by Barbara B. Sherwin, Ph.D., of McGill University in Montreal, Canada, set out to determine whether otherwise healthy surgically menopausal women would experience a decrease in cognitive functioning if they were not treated with hormones postoperatively.

Fifty women were randomly assigned to a group that received either estrogen, an androgen (a hormone that supports masculine characteristics), a combined estrogen/androgen preparation, or a placebo (no hormones). Hormone levels were monitored, and psychological tests were administered pre- and postoperatively. The psychological tests measured short-term memory, long-term memory, and logical reasoning.

The results showed that women who had their ovaries removed and who received the placebo had lower scores on all measures of cognitive functioning postoperatively. These results coincided with their significantly lower blood levels of estradiol and testosterone. The control group, which consisted of women who had hysterectomies but were left with their ovaries intact, showed stability in both their hormone levels and their cognitive functioning.[3]

Research by Bruce McEwen, Ph.D., of Rockefeller University in New York, suggests that estrogen and progesterone regulate the creation and breakdown of synaptic connections (junctions between nerve cells) in laboratory rats whose ovaries have been removed. The absence of estrogen decreases the number of synapses and affects the brain's neurotransmitters (the chemicals that assist in the transmission of impulses between nerves).[4] Estrogen—and its absence—is believed to have a similar effect in humans.

Despite research findings such as Sherwin's and McEwen's, the relationship between cognition and hormonal insufficiency remains controversial because the research is contradictory. Perhaps the inconsistent results stem from the lack of standardization in how the research is performed. For example, Barbara Sherwin points out that in these studies, different hormonal preparations and dosages are used, serum hormone levels are not always monitored, naturally and surgically menopausal women are lumped together, and tests used to measure cognitive functioning differ.[5]

As research continues, it is important to keep in mind that changes in mental functioning are related to performance, not intelligence. You have not suddenly become stupid. And if you are a candidate for estrogen, these changes appear to be reversible with the restoration of adequate amounts of the hormone.

It also must be kept in mind that these changes may be related to other physiological processes that have yet to be determined. Linda, a 44-year-old social worker, and Anna, a 43-year-old accountant, who both had their ovaries removed at the time of their hysterectomies, described their cognitive changes as "blocking on words while talking" and being "unable to retain and recall information."

Irritability, mood swings, anxiety, and depression also can have a profound impact on your personal and professional life. They can create an inner turmoil that eats away at you while at the same time alienating your family, friends, and colleagues. Often, women feel as if they are ready to snap. A survey published in *Midlife Woman* reported that 33 percent of the respondents cited psychological symptoms as their reason for beginning hormone replacement therapy.[6] This should convince you that you are not alone.

Alone is exactly how *HEIDI*, a 32-year-old attorney, felt. Due to a rampant pelvic infection, she had developed an abscess in each of her fallopian tubes, as well as scar tissue throughout her pelvis. She opted for the hysterectomy with both ovaries removed that her physician recommended. Ever since the surgery, she said she felt like she was on "an emotional roller coaster."

Although she had some difficulty with vaginal dryness, night sweats, and dry skin, Heidi's most troubling problem was mood swings. Her emotions ran high and could change from one minute to the next. To make matters worse, she would fly off the handle with her friends and coworkers without really knowing why. It was a very alienating feeling.

Even though Heidi wasn't very troubled by vaginal dryness, night sweats, or dry skin, I still addressed these issues with her. She opted for an estrogen-based vaginal cream, estrogenic herbs, and changes in her sleeping environment to control her symptoms. Additionally, Heidi was single and childless. Upon discussing this issue in detail, we determined that her mood swings were probably aggravated by feelings of grief over the loss of fertility. Therefore, I recommended psychological counseling to help her work through these issues.

———◦•◦———

The debate continues over whether a correlation exists between sudden menopause and emotional health, despite self-reports by countless women and some well-documented research. A study conducted by D. H. Richards and published in *The Lancet* demonstrated that women who have had hysterectomies are four times more likely to become depressed within 3 years of surgery, compared to women who did not undergo the surgery. Specifically, 55 percent of women below the age of 40 experienced postoperative depression.[7] Richards also compared a group of 56 women who had undergone hysterectomies in the previous 5 years with a group of 56 women who had undergone other types of surgery. He found that 70 percent of the women with hysterectomies suffered from depression within 3 years of the surgery, compared to 30 percent of the women who had had other surgery.[8]

According to a report in *Midlife Woman*, estrogen seems to have a "mental tonic" effect and has been shown to relieve depressive feelings in women not suffering from clinical depression.[9]

Often, changes in mood are attributed to circumstances surrounding the sudden menopause or other problems stemming from it. For example, coping with issues such as loss of fertility, a perceived loss of femininity, aging, and the presence of disease can understandably lead to emotional changes. However, these issues do not exist for all women having difficulty with mood swings, anxiety, and depression. Further complicating the situation is the fact that these circumstances also can aggravate a preexisting depression, not necessarily cause it. Determining the cause of depression—hormones versus external factors—is vital to treating it.

Exactly how does the lack of hormones regulate psychological and cognitive functioning? It has been suggested that the mechanism involves the neurotransmitting chemicals that are crucial to neuropsychological functioning. Examples include acetylcholine, norepinephrine, dopamine, and serotonin. In one of Barbara Sherwin's studies, she cites research involving the link between memory, acetylcholine, and estrogen. It seems that giving estradiol supplements to rats whose ovaries had been removed raised the level of acetylcholine.[10]

In her book *Hysterectomy: Before and After,* Winnifred Cutler presents data that relates depression in women who have undergone hysterectomies to decreased levels of an amino acid called tryptophan and to decreased levels of endorphins.[11] Research into the role of neurotransmitters and their powerful impact on human behavior continues. Much of the data is responsible for the strides made with antidepressant medications, since they work by affecting brain chemicals.

On the flip side of the coin, it is important to note that some women report no noticeable changes in psychological well-being associated with sudden menopause, and some women even state that they feel better. Women who have put up with intense pain or profuse menstrual bleeding may report that their quality of life improves. Once again, the experience is very individualized. Clearly, the link between cognitive and psychological functioning and sudden menopause deserves further exploration.

Coping Strategies

Get a physical.

Have an examination to rule out other physical or emotional reasons for the symptoms you are experiencing. If they are related to an underlying health problem, correcting the problem should improve the situation.

Be easy on yourself.

Recognize that you are having difficulty and that it may take some time to resolve these problems. Berating yourself for your shortcomings will only lead to frustration and make the situation worse.

Seek counseling.

Seek counseling for significant anxiety, depression, or stress.

Accentuate the positive in your life.

Try not to dwell on bothersome situations or events that you cannot control. Instead, focus on those areas of your life that you can improve. It also helps to appreciate your blessings.

Look at your medications.

If you are taking medication, talk to your doctor or pharmacist about side effects and/or interactions with food or other medicines. A drug interaction could cause impaired memory or altered mood.

Get an adequate amount of rest.

Fatigue can aggravate irritability and anxiety and impair mental functioning.

Use memory tricks.

Make the most of your memory by utilizing "tricks" to make learning and remembering easier. Try the following tips:

- Engage in activities that stimulate your mind. Do not avoid learning situations because you are afraid that you cannot do it.

- To facilitate information storage and retrieval, repeat several times the information that you want to remember. For example, when you are introduced to someone, immediately say the person's name aloud, then repeat it to yourself several times as you look at the person.

- Discuss current events with friends and family as a way of retaining what you have learned.

- Use "chunking" to group information into manageable amounts. For example, to recall the number 8301200, think about it this way: people begin work at 8:30 and break for lunch at 12:00.

- Relate new information to something else that you already know.

- Think of creative ways to recall information. Remember this rhyme from school: "In 1492, Columbus sailed the ocean blue."

- Write things down.

- Give yourself extra time to learn information.

- Remain as independent as you can, and take care of your own affairs. Being totally dependent on someone else can lead to a lazy mind.

Practice stress-management techniques.

Find stress-management techniques that work for you, and practice them. It is believed that protracted stress can impair learning and memory, as well as aggravate irritability and anxiety. Stress-management techniques include breathing exercises, guided imagery, meditation, and yoga.

Exercise.

Anyone who exercises regularly knows that it not only helps to manage stress, but it enhances well-being and increases self-image. It also improves blood flow to the brain.

Watch Your Diet.

- Follow the Food Guide Pyramid (see Figure 7.1) to ensure a nutritious and well-balanced diet. Brain function relies heavily on adequate nutrition.

- Eat at regular intervals and do not skip meals.

- Maintain an adequate protein intake. As a general rule, you should get 15 to 20 grams per meal. Keep in mind that soy products are good sources of protein. Since soy products are thought to stabilize hormone levels, they may help mood and cognitive changes.

- Avoid large amounts of refined sugar. Doing so helps to equalize your blood-sugar level so you don't feel tired, cranky, and fuzzy-minded.

- Moderate your caffeine intake. While caffeine is a mental stimulant, high doses have the opposite effect.

- Keep your fat intake to less than 30 percent of your total calories. However, do not compulsively eliminate fat from your diet, because dietary fat is necessary for body function, particularly for hormone production.

Experiment with supplements.

Take the time to learn how vitamins, minerals, and herbs work. Also learn their potential side effects and contraindications. The following is a list of supplements for promoting mental and emotional stability and well-being. Supplements are discussed in greater detail in Chapter 5.

vitamin B complex

lecithin

phosphatidylserine

choline

vitamin C

calcium

bioflavonoids

omega-3 fatty acids

L-tyrosine

L-phenylalanine

ginkgo

black cohosh*

St. John's wort

ginseng*

valerian

kava-kava

chamomile

* contains phytoestrogens, which produce estrogen-like effects

Consider medication.

Prescribing hormone replacement therapy to alter mood or enhance mental functioning is controversial. Some women find significant relief; others do not. If you think that your problems are related to a hormone deficiency and if you are a candidate for hormones, talk to your doctor about a trial period to determine if hormones may be helpful (see Chapter 6).

An antianxiety agent or an antidepressant may be suggested if you suffer from significant anxiety or depression. If you have exhausted all other avenues of treatment, you may find one of these medicines to be beneficial. It is important that you are watched carefully by a qualified physician and that you receive appropriate counseling in conjunction with the medicine.

Wrinkles, Weight Gain, and Weariness

"My skin seems drier and less supple. I think it makes me look older." These were the comments of *NOREEN*, a 35-year-old hair-stylist. Being in the cosmetology business, Noreen was very conscious of the changes in her skin and hair that had come about since she had undergone a hysterectomy with BSO.

Following the surgery, she had pelvic radiation to treat uterine cancer. She tried to discuss her concerns with the oncologist, but he was more focused on monitoring her for a recurrence of the cancer. She encountered the same type of response from her family doctor. Soon she began to feel foolish for being bothered by her dry skin and thinning hair, even though these issues were important to her.

In the end, Noreen was able to significantly rehydrate her skin by drinking more water, eliminating alcohol and caffeine, and replacing her facial and body soap with a cleansing cream and shower gel. She also began using a medicated shampoo to stimulate hair growth.

Developing dry skin, adding a few pounds, or getting less sleep might seem inconsequential, but such changes, commonly reported by postmenopausal women, can have a profound impact on well-being and self-esteem. Since they are normally associated with aging, they may be particularly distressing to a sudden menopausal woman in her twenties or thirties. They serve as reminders of the ways in which our bodies respond to hormonal changes. It is understandable how these nonspecific complaints can be attributed to a variety of physical and emotional struggles, as well as to the aging process itself.

During the reproductive years, a woman's hormone levels are at their peak and her skin is in its prime. In general, the skin is thicker, oilier, firmer, and more flexible. This benefit of youth is largely due to the connective tissues collagen and elastin. As we age, the connective tissue gradually breaks down, and the skin becomes drier, thinner, and looser. Wrinkles become more apparent, and fat and muscle tissue begin shrinking.

You also may find that, as you age, your scalp hair becomes thinner, and your facial hair and chest hair become more coarse and noticeable. This is believed to be caused by an imbalance between the estrogens and the androgens, a hormonal imbalance that can make a person appear older than her years.

American women report an increase in body weight with age, and many indicate that the increase began at or near menopause. Is this weight gain a factor of age, hormones, or both?

The relationship between menopause and weight gain is unclear. Some women gain weight and others do not. Most studies conclude that weight gain seems to be more related to metabolic changes associated with aging than to hormonal status. However, when the endocrine system—which produces hormones—is in flux, as happens severely and quickly following sudden menopause, it can drastically influence weight. Some studies do suggest that lack of ovarian function may increase food intake. Along these lines, it is interesting to note that postmenopausal women no longer experience the slight increase in metabolism that occurs during the luteal phase of the menstrual cycle.

Regardless of weight gain, after menopause a woman's body shape may change as the distribution of weight shifts. Breasts and hips tend to lose some fatty tissue, while the upper torso tends to find it. Perhaps the first sign of this migratory pattern of fat is that your clothes fit differently. Also, as we age, our total body fat increases while our muscle mass decreases.

SANDY, a 50-year-old payroll clerk, was diagnosed with breast cancer. She had a mastectomy, underwent chemotherapy, and then was placed on Tamoxifen to induce a medical menopause. In working with her, we were able to decrease the frequency and severity of her hot flashes through dietary changes and the use of supplements, but her greatest area of frustration centered on her weight.

Although she had always been above her ideal body weight, she said that she had "more of a weight problem now." Her overall weight remained about the same, but her body shape changed. She went from being pear shaped to being apple shaped. She also noticed that the weight seemed more stubborn, and she required a more rigorous exercise program to take it off. Sandy eventually was able to lose weight and increase her fitness level, but it required a dedicated effort.

———•◦•———

Some of this weight shifting is attributed to the changing balance between estrogen and testosterone. A lower level of estrogen compared to testosterone tends to tip the scales in the androgenic direction. This may result in changes such as increased facial hair, increased libido, a deepened voice, and "male" distribution of body weight. When the normal ratio of estrogen to testosterone is restored, Mother Nature kicks back in. The good news is that regular exercise has proven to be effective in keeping postmenopausal weight gain at a minimum.

Are you having trouble falling asleep? Do you awaken in the middle of the night or too early in the morning? If so, you are not alone. Disturbances in sleep patterns may occur after sudden menopause.

Often, insomnia is attributed to night sweats. While it is true that temperature changes will interrupt your sleep, there may be other factors at work as well. For example, in addition to its role in temperature regulation, the hypothalamus also plays a role in controlling sleep patterns and is sensitive to changing hormone levels. Recall from Chapter 1 that the endocrine system works as a team; changes in one area may generate changes in another.

"I have not had a restful night's sleep in a while," *SUE* told me. After undergoing a lumpectomy with radiation for breast cancer, Sue, a 41-year-old banker, was placed on Tamoxifen. As a result of her sudden menopause, she was grappling with sleep issues.

After talking to her in some detail, I could see that there were probably several factors at work. She was experiencing some anxiety related to her medical problems and was unable to relax sufficiently at bedtime. I also suspected that her body might be undergoing mild temperature changes at night that didn't fully register with her as she awoke. And of course, there is always that elusive melatonin link when it comes to insomnia. Melatonin is a hormone produced by the pineal gland in the brain. It is responsible for our sleep-wake cycle, and its levels diminish as we age. It is difficult to determine if sleep problems are related to melatonin levels, estrogen levels, or both.

After a few months of listening to relaxation tapes at bedtime, attending a breast cancer support group, and following some of the other suggestions in this chapter, the quality of Sue's sleep improved. Occasionally, she relies on sleep-inducing herbs, but most nights she doesn't need them.

———◆———

No matter what causes it, persistent insomnia results in sleep deprivation, in part from inadequate REM sleep. The REM (rapid eye movement) portion of the sleep cycle takes place when dreaming occurs; it is necessary for the brain cells to rejuvenate themselves. If you fail to get adequate REM sleep, you will feel fatigued and mentally sluggish.

Whether changes in skin, weight, or sleep patterns are due to hormonal imbalances, other health problems, lifestyle, or a combination of these factors, steps can be taken to provide some relief. As with any other symptoms that can occur with a sudden menopause, if they are affecting the quality of your life, then you owe it to yourself to explore treatment options.

Coping Strategies: Dry Skin

▧ Avoid foods and/or activities that dehydrate the skin, particularly alcohol, caffeine, diuretics, dry air, and saunas.

▨ Use a humidifier if you live in a dry climate.

▨ Drink plenty of water to hydrate your system from the inside out.

▨ Limit sun exposure, and use a broad-spectrum sunscreen (one that shields you from both UVA and UVB rays) with a sun protection factor (SPF) of at least 15.

▨ Wash with a super-fatted soap. Consider using a cleansing cream on your face and neck.

▨ Avoid excessive bathing.

▨ Moisturize. This helps to seal in water, especially after washing your face. For daytime use, you can apply a moisturizer that contains sunscreen and deal with two concerns at the same time.

▨ Use oil-based cosmetics. Try to avoid powder blush or loose powder, which can accentuate wrinkles.

▨ Quit smoking.

▨ Get plenty of rest.

▨ Exercise regularly. Exercise improves circulation to the skin.

▨ Eat a well-balanced diet. If you are on a weight-loss program, lose weight slowly. Keep your fat intake to less than 30 percent of your total calories, but do not compulsively eliminate fat from your diet. Essential fatty acids are needed to keep the skin supple. Vitamin C also is needed because it plays a role in collagen synthesis.

▨ Consider medication. If you are a candidate for hormones and are taking them for other reasons, you may delight in the way that your skin responds to them. The hormones help the skin to stay oilier, thicker, and more elastic. Estrogen supports the oil glands, fat tissue, and connective tissue. However, in some women, estrogen and testosterone can lead to acne (see Chapter 6).

Coping Strategies: Weight Gain

- Keep a 3-day food log so that you can evaluate what you are eating and the amount you are eating. Do not cheat. If it goes into your mouth, it goes into your food log.

- Follow the Food Guide Pyramid (see Chapter 7). This will ensure a balanced diet of nutrient-rich food.

- Do not starve yourself. When you do, your metabolism actually slows down further to compensate for the drastic reduction in calories.

- Limit the number of calories from fat to less than 30 percent of your total daily intake. For the average woman, 44 grams of fat per day is sufficient. Also, gradually increase your intake of dietary fiber. Consuming 25 to 35 grams of fiber per day is desirable for most women.

- Attend cooking classes or nutrition classes that teach you how to modify your recipes for tasty, low-fat meals. Try to find classes that provide taste testing and recipes.

- Consider nutrition counseling with a registered dietitian if you are having difficulty managing your weight. Bring your 3-day food log so that the dietitian can assess your food intake.

- Seek the help of a specialist in eating disorders and a registered dietitian if you engage in starvation dieting, binge-purge eating, or compulsive overeating. This is especially essential if extreme weight loss from an eating disorder is the cause of your sudden menopause. If changes in your appetite are related to depression, seek therapy.

- Get moving! Increase your daily activity level. For example, climb a few flights of stairs rather than take the elevator, walk more and drive less, and get things yourself instead of sending your children for them.

◈ Exercise for at least 30 to 45 minutes most days of the week. Alternate between aerobic and muscle-toning activities. Aerobic exercise burns calories, and muscle toning boosts metabolism. If an exercise professional is designing a fitness program for you, ask about a body-fat composition analysis. This gives a breakdown of the percentage of fat, muscle, and water in your body. Such information is helpful in developing an exercise program to meet your specific needs.

◈ Avoid appetite suppressants. Neither over-the-counter nor prescription medicines help to teach the lifelong habits that are necessary for long-term weight loss.

Coping Strategies: Insomnia

◈ Establish regular sleep patterns. Go to bed and awaken at the same time each day.

◈ Preserve your body's melatonin supply by allowing sunlight into your bedroom in the morning to wake you, minimizing your light exposure 1 to 2 hours before bedtime, and avoiding night-shift work.

◈ If night sweats are keeping you from a good night's rest, take measures to control them.

◈ Keep your bedroom at a comfortable temperature or even slightly cool.

◈ Learn to associate your bed with sleep (and sex, of course). Do not engage in activities such as eating, reading, or watching TV in bed.

◈ Daily exercise is beneficial in dealing with insomnia. However, avoid exercising within 2 to 3 hours of bedtime; doing so will invigorate you and make it difficult to fall asleep.

- Do not review the day's events or plan tomorrow's activities at bedtime. Allot time for this at least 2 hours before retiring.

- Try not to become fixated on your inability to sleep. Instead, focus on relaxing.

- If drinking warm milk before bedtime works for you, do it. Milk contains a chemical called tryptophan, which is believed to induce relaxation. However, frequent trips to the bathroom can disrupt sleep, too.

- Avoid stimulants such as caffeinated beverages, some pain relievers, nasal decongestants, cold and sinus medicine, appetite suppressants, and antidepressants at bedtime.

- Avoid using alcohol. It interferes with the sleep cycle so that your sleep is not as restful. You also can develop a dependency on alcohol.

- Use relaxation strategies to help you drift off to sleep. Examples include progressive muscle relaxation, soothing music, or visualization.

- Seek evaluation for persistent insomnia to rule out an underlying medical disorder. Keep in mind that anxiety and depression can manifest themselves through insomnia. Seek therapy for these disorders.

- Consider consulting a specialist in sleep disorders.

- Experiment with nutritional supplements, after you have become knowledgeable about how vitamins, minerals, and herbs work. Be sure to consider their potential side effects and contraindications. Following are the names of some supplements that may aid insomnia. Supplements are discussed in greater detail in Chapter 5.

valerian

kava-kava

chamomile

balm

celery

hop

motherwort

passion flower

skullcap

yarrow

- If night sweats are the cause of your insomnia and you are a candidate for estrogen, you will probably find significant relief with estrogen therapy. Another benefit of estrogen is that it is thought to restore REM sleep, which leads to a better night's rest. This is discussed in greater detail in Chapter 6.

- Medications are commonly prescribed for insomnia. If you are considering using a medication, learn all you can about it, and consult a pharmacist. Tranquilizers and other sleep aids can be habit forming. Over-the-counter sleep aids typically contain antihistamines, which have sleep-inducing properties. Occasional use is not harmful, but sleep aids should not be relied upon regularly.

Chapter Highlights

- Remember that a sudden menopause is more immediate and severe than a natural menopause. Therefore, it may require more time and more coping strategies for resolving some of your menopausal changes.

- Even though the changes you are experiencing are most likely due to depletion of your ovarian hormones, it is a good idea to start with a general physical exam. Depending on your symptoms, this may also include some blood work or other tests that your doctor deems necessary. Remember, the endocrine hormones work as a team, so an imbalance in one area can result in an imbalance in another area. A physical will help to rule out an underlying medical condition that could be contributing to your situation.

◎ After consulting the list of coping strategies for the menopausal changes you are experiencing, choose one or two suggestions that you think you can most benefit from. Every few weeks, reevaluate how you are feeling and decide if you should add one or two more.

◎ Be sure to consult the chapters on dietary supplements and hormone replacement therapy if you choose these options. At the end of Chapter 5, you will find a chart that provides specific guidelines for treating menopausal changes using supplements. There also is more direction on using soy in the chapter titled "Creating Health."

◎ Do not become discouraged. You will feel better. Talk to other women who have experienced a sudden menopause and find out what worked for them. This exchange of ideas may steer you in the right direction.

Doc Talk

◎ Make sure to impress upon your doctor the importance of your daily quality of life.

◎ Be honest with your physician about the menopausal changes you are experiencing. Ask if she or he has read about anything that could help. If your doctor is unable to help you, request a referral to someone who can.

◎ When you hit upon coping strategies that work for you, communicate them to your physician. You never know when your experience will help another patient.

3

Building Better Bones

"I'm not really concerned about osteoporosis because it doesn't run in my family," said MAUREEN, a 47-year-old housewife. At age 45, Maureen underwent a hysterectomy with BSO because of uterine fibroids and endometriosis. She tried using various forms of estrogen, but found that they aggravated her migraine headaches. Therefore, she stopped taking the hormone. Despite her low lifetime intake of calcium and her sudden menopause with its resulting loss of estrogen, she did not perceive osteoporosis as a threat to her health because she did not have osteoporosis in her family history.

I gave her a few pamphlets to read on the risk factors and development of osteoporosis. Soon thereafter, she underwent a bone density test, which revealed that she had weak bones for her age. She is now taking calcium, vitamin D, and magnesium, as well as engaging in weight-bearing exercise 5 days a week, in hopes of slowing down the bone loss. In 2 years, she will undergo another bone density test to gauge the effectiveness of these actions.

———•◦•———

One of the most prevalent misconceptions I encounter as a women's health educator is that if there is no family history of osteoporosis, a woman does not need to be concerned. This can be a dangerous attitude.

Every woman should be taking steps right now to prevent osteoporosis from being a part of her future. However, doing so is particularly important for those who have experienced sudden menopause. The loss of ovarian functioning—and the resulting loss of hormones—is a significant risk factor for bone demineralization. Sudden menopausal women, since they are often younger than women who undergo natural menopause, especially cannot afford to ignore this issue, because they potentially face more years of hormonal shortages and therefore more years of bone loss. Making an investment in your bones now will result in big dividends in your future quality of life.

Osteoporosis: The Silent Thief

The word osteoporosis literally means porous bone. It is a debilitating condition in which bones become fragile, lose their strength, and break. You may hear osteoporosis referred to as the "silent thief," because it develops over the course of several years without any outward signs. It can progress undetected for decades.

Typically, women do not ingest enough daily calcium over their lifetime, but the consequences of their actions do not become apparent until midlife or beyond. Bones depend upon calcium for strength. Perhaps surprisingly, bones are living tissue. They are constantly being remodeled because of wear and tear. Bone cells called osteoclasts break down bone, and cells called osteoblasts make new bone.

Maximum bone density occurs between 25 and 35 years of age. After that time, bone loss slowly exceeds bone formation as osteoclast activity outpaces osteoblast activity. Sudden menopause at any age can be damaging to the bones, but the younger the woman who experiences sudden menopause, the more devastating the potential for bone loss.

If the bone loss becomes excessive, bones become less dense, and fractures (breaks) occur. Any lifting action, fall, or blow to a bone that normally would not cause a problem can result in a break. The most common sites for breaks include the hips, wrists, and spine. Spinal fractures also can result in a loss of height and a dowager's hump (stooped posture).

If you are still not convinced that osteoporosis can be a serious health threat for women, consider the following facts:

- Women can lose up to 20 percent of their total bone mass in the first 5 to 7 years following menopause.[1]

- More than 25 million Americans—mostly women—are at high risk for developing osteoporosis, yet a Gallup survey of women ages 45 to 75 indicates that three out of four women have never spoken to their doctors about the disease.[2]

- Osteoporosis leads to 1.5 million fractures each year.[3]

- One in three women older than 50 will suffer a vertebral fracture. Vertebral fractures can cause the spine to collapse and lead to a loss of height and stooped posture.[4]

- A woman's risk of developing a hip fracture is equal to her combined risk of developing breast, uterine, and ovarian cancers.[5]

- Osteoporosis can cause crippling, painful, lasting disability.

Prevention and Early Detection

ELIZABETH is a 68-year-old retiree who had a hysterectomy with BSO 25 years ago due to uterine fibroids. At the time of her surgery, she reported frequent daily hot flashes and night sweats so severe that her husband "thought I was nuts because I was up at night opening the windows." However, she did not consider estrogen as an option. She said that over the years she and her doctor did not discuss estrogen therapy. When I asked her if she had been taking preventive measures to thwart the development of osteoporosis, she replied, "I didn't think osteoporosis was an issue for me. I just don't think about it."

Elizabeth talked to her doctor about her newfound concerns. He ordered a bone density test, and she was shocked to discover that she had severe osteopenia (bone loss that precedes osteoporosis). She was started on medicine to stimulate new bone growth and prevent fractures.

———•◦•———

Not only is osteoporosis preventable, if it is present and detected early, further bone loss can be dramatically reduced. To protect yourself from the ravages of osteoporosis, you must be able to identify the factors that increase your risk of developing the disease. To determine your risk, answer yes or no to the following questions:[6]

- Do you have a small, thin frame, or are you Caucasian or Asian?

- Has a female member of your immediate family broken a bone as an adult?

- Are you a postmenopausal woman?

- Have you had an early or surgically induced menopause?

- Have you been taking high doses of thyroid medication, or high or prolonged doses of cortisone-like drugs for asthma, arthritis, or cancer?

- Is your diet low in dairy products and other sources of calcium?

- Are you physically inactive?

- Do you smoke cigarettes or drink alcohol in excess?

The more times you answered "yes," the greater your risk of developing osteoporosis. A few of these risk factors—such as gender and family history—cannot be changed. However, several of the risks for osteoporosis involve lifestyle choices and are thus modifiable. Let's take a closer look at each of these risk factors and at how they influence bone formation and bone loss.

Gender—Although men develop osteoporosis, it is far more common in women. This can be attributed to our smaller bone mass, postmenopausal hormone decline, and penchant for compulsive dieting.

Build—Women with small frames have less bone mass and cannot afford to lose much of it. Women with extremely low percentages of body fat do not store estrogen as efficiently and might even stop ovulating, which inhibits progesterone production. Hormones are very influential in the process of building bone.

Race—Osteoporosis is more prevalent in Caucasian and Asian women (especially those who do not eat a traditional Asian diet). However, African American and Hispanic women are still at significant risk.

Heredity—If you have relatives with osteoporosis or dowagers' humps, who are susceptible to fractures, or who have lost height, your risk is increased. This may be related to body structure. Another theory regarding hereditary osteoporosis correlates a defective vitamin D receptor gene with the development of bone loss, since vitamin D is needed to absorb calcium.

Menopause—A sudden or early menopause leaves your bones vulnerable for a longer period of time. Estrogen is vital for maximum absorption of calcium. New studies also reveal the important roles that progesterone and testosterone play in building bone. After menopause, hormone levels decline. Since the ovaries are the powerhouses of hormone production, removal of the ovaries is even more devastating to the bones unless hormone replacement therapy is initiated.

Medication—Prolonged use of certain medicines can affect calcium absorption and excretion. These medicines include glucocorticoids (anti-inflammatory drugs such as cortisone and prednisone), anticonvulsants (seizure medicine), diuretics (water pills), and antacids. High doses of thyroid hormone also can affect calcium absorption. If you are on any maintenance medication, ask your doctor or pharmacist if the medicine is known to affect bone loss.

Lack of calcium—A diet low in calcium can have a profound effect on the development of osteoporosis. Calcium is discussed in further detail later in this chapter.

Physical inactivity—Regular, weight-bearing exercise is necessary for building and maintaining strong bones. Walking, jogging, hiking, racquet sports, weight lifting, aerobics, and stair climbing are all considered weight-bearing exercise, because they force you to work against gravity. At least 30 minutes of exercise five to six times per week is most beneficial.

Smoking—Smoking depletes the body of nutrients, including calcium, and decreases estrogen levels.

Alcohol—Excessive alcohol consumption can impair calcium absorption.

Diet—Protein is an important part of our daily diet. However, high-protein diets do facilitate calcium excretion. As a general rule, adequate daily protein intake is .8 grams per kilogram of body weight. The average recommended daily allowance (RDA) of protein for women is 50 grams.

In addition, there is evidence that a diet high in caffeine and carbonated beverages inhibits the availability of calcium. Many women tend to substitute caffeinated or carbonated beverages for milk in their daily diet.

Gray hair and false teeth—No, your eyes are not deceiving you. According to Trevor Stamp's study, "Gray Hair, False Teeth and Bad Bones," men and women with premature gray hair (50 percent gray by the age of 40) are 4.4 times more likely to have weak bones. However, more research is needed to verify this link. Also, several studies have shown a correlation between total bone mass and tooth loss. Bone resorption may result in mandibular (jaw) changes, which can lead to tooth loss.

Diagnosis and Treatment

After you and your doctor have carefully assessed your risk factors and medical history, you may decide to have your bone mass measured. There are various diagnostic tests that can be used, all of which are simple, noninvasive, and painless radiographic techniques. These tests use small amounts of radiation to determine the density of the bones in the hip, spine, wrist, and heel. Routine X rays are not sensitive enough to detect changes until 20 percent to 30 percent of bone tissue is lost.[7]

Of all the bone density tests, dual-energy X-ray absorptiometry (DEXA) is considered the gold standard in the diagnosis of osteoporosis. It can measure virtually any skeletal bone, and it is very quick and accurate. It has the added bonus of being quite precise. In other words, it can measure miniscule changes in bone density from year to year, while emitting minimal radiation (much less than a standard chest X ray).

Sadly, many insurance companies will not pay for this test unless a woman meets specific criteria. Medicare recently began covering this test for women ages 65 and older. Since the goal is to prevent osteoporosis by detecting early signs of bone loss (osteopenia), oftentimes it is too late to begin testing at age 65. The current insurance criteria exclude those very women who, unbeknownst to them and their doctors, are losing bone and are at risk for osteoporosis. This definitely includes women who have undergone sudden menopause. That is why I believe that all sudden menopausal women should be screened by bone mineral density testing.

In conjunction with poor insurance reimbursement, the cost of obtaining a DEXA scan usually prohibits its use as a screening tool. However, peripheral DEXA scans tend to be more economical and are accurate enough to make them a good choice for screening purposes.

The peripheral DEXA scan measures the mass of the heel or wrist to give an indication if the density is normal, osteopenic, or osteoporotic. If the results of the test are abnormal, that scan should be followed up with a central DEXA for confirmation and monitoring.

Another diagnostic tool that is now being used in the same way as the peripheral DEXA is ultrasound. With ultrasound, bone density is estimated according to the way sound waves penetrate the bone. The equipment used to perform peripheral DEXA and ultrasound exams is portable, increasing the accessibility of what I consider to be a very vital screening for most women.

New urine tests have been developed to assess the risk of osteoporosis and to monitor the effectiveness of drug therapy. An example of this is Pyrilinks, which detects the presence of bone collagen in the urine. Increased levels of bone collagen indicate accelerated bone resorption (excretion). However, bone mineral testing remains more accurate.

Existing 24-hour urine tests that can screen for potential bone loss involve calculating the ratio of calcium to creatinine and of calcium to hydroxyproline (the same substance tested for in the Pyrilinks test). This ratio indicates the rate of calcium excretion.

Currently, a doctor's order is needed for all of these laboratory and diagnostic tests. Be sure to discuss the advantages, disadvantages, radiation exposure, and cost of each test method with your doctor.

The results of your bone density test may indicate the need for medication to help stop further bone loss and prevent fractures. Although no cure exists for osteoporosis, the use of medication can help to maintain bone mass and significantly alter the progression of this condition. In preliminary studies, a few of these medications have been shown to actually rebuild bone.

When combined with an adequate daily calcium intake, hormone supplementation has proven to be the single most effective method for preventing osteoporosis. Estrogen works by helping your bones absorb and retain calcium to inhibit the breakdown of bone cells. Recently, the roles of progesterone, progestin, and testosterone in combating osteoporosis have stimulated great interest, as they appear to foster bone-cell generation. However, not everyone wants or is a candidate for hormone replacement therapy.

Calcitonin is another hormone that has been approved by the Food and Drug Administration to treat osteoporosis. In its natural form, calcitonin is produced by the thyroid gland to help regulate calcium levels. Injectable salmon calcitonin regimens (synthetically manufactured to replicate the structure of salmon calcitonin; it does not come from salmon) have proven to increase bone mass and can be continued indefinitely. An adequate calcium intake also is required.

Side effects of calcitonin therapy have included skin rash, flushing of the face and hands, nausea, and urinary frequency. Calcitonin also is available as a nasal spray (Miacalcin). The most common complaints of this therapy are a runny nose and nasal irritation. Since using a nasal spray is more appealing than getting injections, the popularity of this approach to therapy is skyrocketing, and the injectable form is not commonly used.

Bisphosphonates are another class of medicines that are used in the treatment of osteoporosis. Etidronate (Didronel) is given in an intermittent, cyclical fashion daily for 2 weeks, repeated every 3 months. This drug is taken orally, on an empty stomach. Sufficient calcium is required, but if supplementation is needed, calcium and etidronate should not be taken together.[8] Side effects of etidronate include nausea and diarrhea.[9] Although etidronate appears to increase bone mass, it has not been proven to reduce bone fractures.

Another bisphosphonate—alendronate (Fosamax)—recently has gained approval from the FDA for the prevention and treatment of osteoporosis. It can be used alone or in combination with estrogen to inhibit bone demineralization. Additionally, two new studies demonstrate that alendronate prevents bone loss in menopausal women with low bone mass.[10] An adequate intake of calcium is helpful to this process.

It is imperative that alendronate be taken daily on an empty stomach. The manufacturer recommends taking it in the morning with a glass of water, and waiting at least 30 minutes before eating or drinking anything else. To minimize gastric reflux, it is recommended that you do not lie down for at least 30 minutes after taking alendronate. The most commonly reported side effects of alendronate are digestive disturbances.

A third bisphosphonate—risedronate (Actonel)—recently has gained FDA approval for the prevention and treatment of osteoporosis. The dosing restrictions, instructions for use, and occurrence of side effects are similar to those for Fosamax.

The use of fluorides in the treatment of osteoporosis is being investigated but remains controversial. In high doses, fluorides stimulate new bone growth, but the new tissue is structurally different from and weaker than normal bone. It also is crucial that appropriate intakes of calcium and vitamin D be ensured. However, in a randomized, placebo-controlled trial of 110 women with postmenopausal osteoporosis, slow-release sodium fluoride given twice daily in four 14-month cycles (12 months on, 2 months off) along with 400 mg of calcium citrate twice daily increased spinal bone mass. Side effects of this therapy included minor gastrointestinal irritation.[11]

The newest class of drugs that have received FDA approval for treatment of osteoporosis is the "selective estrogen receptor modulators." Referred to as "designer estrogens," these drugs mimic the effects of estrogen on the bones—and on the heart (see Chapter 4)—without stimulating breast or uterine tissue. The only drawback of these drugs is that they do not halt hot flashes; in fact, they may aggravate them.

An example of a designer estrogen is Evista (raloxifene). Evista provides an alternative to hormone replacement therapy for women who are at high risk for osteoporosis or who already have osteoporosis. Evista reduces overall bone turnover and increases bone density while simultaneously decreasing total cholesterol and LDL (bad) cholesterol. Another advantage is that it does not stimulate breast or uterine tissue the way estrogen does.

During the 2½ years of clinical trials for Evista, breast tenderness and spotting were not reported, and risk of breast and uterine cancer did not increase. In fact, incidence of breast cancer decreased by about 50 percent. Keep in mind that because this is a new drug, no long-term details are available. The most frequently reported side effects of Evista were hot flashes and leg cramps. And if you have a history of liver disease or deep-vein thrombosis (blood clots), you are not a candidate for this medicine.

Boning Up on Calcium

"Even though I'm at high risk for osteoporosis, I really don't have to worry about it until I'm much older, right?" asked JO, a 32-year-old drug-and-alcohol counselor. Jo was diagnosed with breast cancer at age 28 and had been subjected to 4 years of various forms of chemotherapy, radiation, and steroid treatment. She also was taking Tamoxifen. While Tamoxifen does not cause the bones to demineralize—in fact, it affords some protection—the other cancer treatments had taken their toll on her bones. When we met, she was seeking help in managing her menopausal symptoms. However, she did not realize that osteoporosis could rear its ugly head at an early age, given her medical history. For that reason, she was paying little attention to her dietary calcium intake and was not taking supplements, nor had she been referred for a bone density test.

Unfortunately, Jo was diagnosed with osteoporosis. Since she was undergoing various forms of cancer treatment at any given time, she was not placed on bone-building medicine. Instead, she took calcium, vitamin D, and magnesium supplements and paid closer attention to her diet. She also took steps to safety-proof her house to prevent falls, which could have resulted in a broken bone.

Do you get enough calcium? According to the National Osteoporosis Foundation, most women consume less than half of the recommended daily requirement of calcium.[12] Although calcium is present in a variety of foods, the most concentrated source of calcium is dairy products, especially milk. Many women assume that they no longer need this vital mineral after they have reached adulthood, so they stop drinking milk. Other reasons for women's insufficient calcium intake include dieting, following a vegan diet (one allowing no animal products at all), lactose intolerance, and allergies.

According to the National Institutes of Health, postmenopausal women taking estrogen require at least 1,000 mg of calcium daily, the same as premenopausal adult women who are not pregnant or lactating. Postmenopausal women not taking estrogen require at least 1,500 mg of calcium daily, as do all women over the age of 65. On the other hand, the DRI (dietary reference intake; see Chapter 5 for a discussion of this term) for these groups of women recently was increased from 800 mg to 1,200 mg daily, regardless of hormone status. Since the recommendations of these sources differ, choose the highest of the recommendations for your age and menopausal status.

These dosages make it difficult for most women to consume enough calcium in their diets alone. The most efficient way to ensure an adequate calcium intake is to obtain as much as you can from food sources and the rest from supplements. Remember, if you do not ingest enough calcium daily, your body will simply rob it from your bones.

Vitamin D also plays an important role in calcium absorption. Without it, calcium cannot be utilized. Most people are able to obtain enough vitamin D because it is present in milk and is synthesized in the skin through exposure to sunlight. Lengthy sunbathing is unnecessary, as studies have shown that 10 to 15 minutes of unprotected sun exposure to the arms and face two to three times a week is sufficient.

Vitamin D supplementation may be needed in the elderly, the housebound, and those at high risk of osteoporosis. Additionally, consider supplementing if you live in a location that has a long rainy season or dark winters. If you can't tolerate milk or don't like it, supplement with 400 to 800 IUs (international units) of vitamin D, which can be consumed in a multiple vitamin or a calcium-vitamin D preparation. Do not exceed 800 IUs without talking to your doctor or nutritionist, because too much vitamin D can be harmful. If you are taking a multivitamin, be sure to consider the amount of vitamin D included in that pill as part of your total daily intake.

Other nutrients besides vitamin D influence calcium absorption and utilization. Magnesium plays a role. Yet a diet high in calcium can prevent absorption of magnesium. This is a highly competitive relationship, and a balance must exist between calcium and magnesium. For that reason, an adequate magnesium intake—300 to 400 mg—is necessary. Natural sources of this element include dairy products, grains, seafood, meat, lima beans, asparagus, avocados, and strawberries. Another option is to take a magnesium supplement or a multivitamin that contains an adequate amount of magnesium.

Dietary Sources

The best way to assess your calcium intake is to keep a 3-day food log. Record everything you ingest, as well as the amounts, then use a nutrient guide to determine the amount of calcium in each item. The results will probably motivate you to incorporate more calcium-rich foods into your diet. This is becoming easier to do, as more foods are being fortified with calcium (orange juice, for example), and more low-fat and nonfat dairy and soy products are now available. If you do not like milk, eat cheese or yogurt.

Vegetarian sources of calcium include broccoli, rhubarb, baked beans, collard greens, and turnip greens. Tofu and other soy products are also good sources. Many green leafy vegetables—such as spinach, beet greens, and Swiss chard—also contain calcium. Keep in mind, however, that calcium from some leafy green vegetables is poorly absorbed because of the presence of oxalic acid. This may translate into minimal calcium benefits. Still, enjoying these nutritious foods is an integral part of maintaining a balanced diet.

The following tables list calcium-rich foods and their nutritional benefits.

Table 3.1: Dairy Foods

Food	Serving Size	Calcium (mg)	Calories	Fat (g)
Skim milk	1 cup	302	86	0.4
1% milk	1 cup	300	102	2.6
Whole milk	1 cup	291	150	8.2
1% cottage cheese	½ cup	69	82	1.2
Cheddar cheese	1 oz.	204	114	9.4
Plain yogurt (low-fat)	8 oz.	400	140	4.0
Vanilla ice milk	½ cup	92	92	2.8
Mozzarella cheese (part skim)	1 oz.	183	72	4.5
Vanilla soft serve	½ cup	138	111	2.3

Table 3.2: Other Foods

Food	Serving Size	Calcium (mg)	Calories	Fat (g)
Soy milk	1 cup	160	130	4.0
Dried apricots	10 halves	37	311	1.0
Raw bok choy	1 cup	74	9	0.0
Broccoli (frozen, chopped, boiled)	½ cup	47	25	0.1
Collard greens (frozen, chopped, boiled)	½ cup	179	31	0.4
Kale (frozen, chopped, boiled)	½ cup	90	20	0.3
Blackstrap molasses	1 tbsp.	172	47	0.0
Boiled navy beans	1 cup	128	259	1.0
Boiled pinto beans	1 cup	82	235	0.9
Canned refried beans	1 cup	118	270	2.7
Pink salmon (canned with bones)	3 oz.	181	118	5.1
Sardines with bones	3 oz.	371	175	11.2
Raw, firm tofu	½ cup	258	183	11.0

Source: Bowes and Church[13]

Lactose Intolerance

A person who has been diagnosed with lactose intolerance has difficulty digesting lactose, the sugar found in milk. In order to fully process lactose, a special enzyme, lactase, is needed. If your body does not manufacture enough lactase, the lactose passes through the body undigested and unabsorbed. This leads to abdominal cramping, bloating, gas, and diarrhea when certain dairy products are consumed or if large portions are eaten.

Everyone's tolerance level is different. If you are lactose intolerant, you may have to make some dietary modifications, but you can still obtain the required amount of calcium through diet and the use of supplements. In addition to the tips below, using soy milk and eating vegetable sources of calcium are beneficial.

Tips for Lactose Intolerance[14]

- Try using special enzyme tablets formulated for people with a lactase deficiency. They make it possible to consume dairy products.

- Buy lactose-reduced or lactose-free milk. It contains about 70 percent less lactose than regular milk. You also can treat regular milk with an enzyme product that breaks down the sugar.

- Consume milk in servings of one cup or less, and drink it with food. Using smaller amounts of milk and combining it with food decrease the likelihood of symptoms.

- Incorporate cheese into your diet. Much of the lactose is removed during processing. Aged, hard cheeses have a lower sugar content.

- Include yogurt with active cultures in your diet. The active cultures digest the lactose.

Calcium Supplements

It is not always possible or feasible to obtain your entire calcium requirement from food. Although you should include calcium-rich foods in your diet on a daily basis, supplements may be needed to reach the recommended daily requirement.

A multitude of calcium supplements exists today. It can be overwhelming and intimidating to stand in front of a display containing dozens of choices. To add to your dilemma, not all of these products are created equal. When selecting a supplement, keep two factors in mind: the amount of elemental calcium and its bioavailability.

What Is Elemental Calcium?

Elemental calcium is the actual amount of calcium in each tablet. In order to manufacture a tablet or liquid supplement, the elemental calcium is combined with a salt to form a chemical compound for the body to use. Examples of such compounds include calcium carbonate, calcium citrate, and calcium gluconate.

Determining the amount of elemental calcium involves scrutinizing the label. The tablet weight includes the total compound; however, the tablet itself contains less elemental calcium. Be sure to find the actual amount of elemental calcium and calculate your requirements accordingly.

Calcium carbonate is the most concentrated source of calcium. Forty percent of the total weight is derived from elemental calcium. In other words, a 500 mg tablet contains 200 mg of elemental calcium. Calcium citrate is 24 percent elemental calcium, calcium citrate malate is 20 percent, and calcium gluconate is 9 percent.

Bioavailability

No matter how much calcium you take, unless it becomes soluble (dissolves) in your stomach and gets into your bloodstream, it is useless. Calcium supplements need stomach acid to dissolve. Ideally, the tablet should be digested by gastric juices so that it is available to be circulated by the blood (bioavailability). This "solubility factor" differs among types and brands of calcium supplements, as well as among different lots of the same brand.

To test how well a tablet disintegrates, place it in a glass of white vinegar for 30 minutes, stirring every 5 minutes. If the tablet dissolves or breaks up in the glass, it should be soluble in your stomach. Remember to perform this test each time you buy a new bottle of supplements, because there is not always consistency within the same brand. However, many brand labels now advertise their adherence to dissolution testing.

Because a normal amount of stomach acid is necessary for maximum bioavailability of calcium, and because stomach-acid secretion decreases with age, women over 50 need special consideration. These women may want to take their supplements with meals, instead of on an empty stomach. During meals, the stomach naturally increases the amount of acid produced. (Actually, it is a good idea for anyone taking supplements to take them with meals.)

Another option for women over 50, as well as for all women with digestive problems, is to take calcium citrate or calcium citrate malate, because these have optimal bioavailability and are easy to digest. The side effects reported with other types of calcium (bloating, gas, and constipation) are less common with calcium citrate or malate. However, since these supplements are not the most concentrated sources of calcium, more tablets are needed to reach the appropriate dosage.

Tips for Taking Calcium

- Calcium is better absorbed when taken with meals. If you are over 50, have a problem with absorption, or find that calcium upsets your stomach, be sure to take it on a full stomach.

- When taking your supplement, drink a large glass of water to promote absorption.

- Do not take more than 500–600 mg of calcium at one time. It is more effective to take smaller doses several times a day.

- Avoid bone meal or dolomite as a source of calcium. They may contain metals, such as lead. However, although testing is optional and at the discretion of the manufacturer because supplements are not regulated like medications, some calcium preparations are tested to ensure that they do not contain significant amounts of metal.[15] In general, the companies that check for the presence of metals advertise the fact that their product is free of them.

- Natural calcium, such as that found in oyster shell, is no more effective than a synthetically formulated supplement, although it may cost more.

- If you have a personal or family history of kidney stones, consult your doctor before taking a calcium supplement. It may be wise for you to try to obtain most of your calcium from dietary sources. If supplemental calcium is needed, try the citrate or citrate malate for greater bioavailability. Getting enough magnesium also may lower the likelihood of kidney stone formation.

Chapter Highlights

- Sudden menopause, with its subsequent loss of ovarian hormones, predisposes a woman to significant bone loss. The most profound loss of bone occurs during the first 5 to 7 years after menopause. For sudden menopausal women, these changes often occur earlier in life than they would with a natural menopause, resulting in significantly more years when her bones are subject to demineralization.

- Keep a food log for 3 days, and then check it against the foods listed in this chapter or in another food guide to determine the average amount of calcium you consume in a day. Subtract that amount from your daily requirement

(1,200–1,500 mg). The difference is what you will need to make up by taking a calcium supplement or by adding more calcium-rich foods to your diet.

- Most women need to take a calcium supplement. Calcium citrate and calcium citrate malate are the most easily absorbed forms of calcium supplements. It is essential that calcium be taken daily. Adding vitamin D and magnesium will enhance the effectiveness of calcium.

- Be sure to engage in regular weight-bearing exercise, which is vital to maintaining strong bones.

Doc Talk

- Evaluate your risk factors for osteoporosis with your doctor. Discuss ways of lowering your risk.

- Talk to your doctor and pharmacist about any medication you might be taking that could deplete your bones. If it is not possible to switch the medicine, be sure your bone density is monitored.

- Ask your doctor about getting a bone mineral density test. If your medical insurance will not cover a DEXA test, consider paying out-of-pocket for a peripheral DEXA test.

- Discuss follow-up bone mineral density testing and the use of medication if the results of your bone density test are abnormal.

4

A Woman's Heart:

Handle with Care

Picture this: it is a cold, blustery winter day. You are walking down the street when you come across someone lying on the sidewalk, clutching their chest and complaining of chest pain. Your immediate thought will likely be, "Oh no, this person is having a heart attack!" Did you picture the person as a man? Most people do, and that is the problem.

This gender bias could be seen in *DONNA*, a 30-year-old laborer. While undergoing chemotherapy for breast cancer, Donna's periods ceased. She began having hot flashes and mood swings, and then she finally put two and two together. She realized she was in menopause. However, she didn't realize that her hormones were also linked to her heart. "I thought men were the ones who had heart attacks," she said.

After assessing Donna's lifestyle, we targeted a few areas that needed to be addressed. Of immediate concern to both of us was that she smoked. Given her increased risk of heart disease as a sudden menopausal woman, not to mention her history of breast cancer, this created a recipe for disaster. Together we identified smoking as the one risk factor that needed to be corrected first. After talking to her doctor, Donna began using a nicotine patch and attending smoking cessation classes.

There is a misconception that prevails among health-care professionals and the public that women do not develop heart disease or die of heart attacks as frequently as men do. This attitude can be deadly. As women, we generally fail to perceive heart disease as a legitimate threat to our health.

KATHY, a 44-year-old lab technician, told me, "When I think of heart disease, I think of my husband, not myself." She held on to this belief even though her uterine cancer necessitated a hysterectomy with BSO and disqualified her from using estrogen.

Fortunately, Kathy was what most people consider to be a "health nut." Even though she didn't realize that she was at an increased risk of heart disease, she was already eating a low-fat, high-fiber diet and maintaining a healthy weight. Regular exercise had been a part of her lifestyle for years. In addition to raising her awareness of how sudden menopause increases a woman's risk of heart disease, I suggested she use vitamin E, coenzyme Q10, and vitamin B complex for cardioprotection.

Perhaps the following facts from the American Heart Association will underscore the gravity of the situation for women in the United States:

- One in nine women aged 45 to 64 has some form of cardiovascular disease. This statistic climbs to one in three for women 65 and older.

- Approximately 6,000 women under age 65 die each year of heart attacks; more than 25 percent of them are under 45.

- Heart disease is even more of a threat for African Americans. The death rate from coronary artery disease is 28 percent higher for black women than it is for white women. From ages 35 to 84, the death rate from heart attacks among black women is 1.4 times that of white women.

- Heart and blood-vessel diseases combined claim the lives of more than 485,000 women each year. That compares with 223,000 deaths from all forms of cancer.

- Of the nearly 500,000 heart-attack deaths each year, about 240,000 are women.[1]

So how did the mistaken perception that women are less susceptible to heart disease come about? Probably because men develop heart disease at a younger age than women—about a decade earlier on average. Premenopausal women seem to be protected by estrogen. Therefore, researchers over the years have mostly studied the "typical heart attack victim": the white, middle-aged male. The results gleaned from these studies were simply extrapolated and applied to women.

We now know, however, that this approach is not always valid. A woman's body responds differently when it comes to the diagnosis and treatment of heart disease. For example, women are more likely than men to die from their first heart attack or to have a subsequent attack. Since females are older when cardiovascular disease develops, they are more likely also to be suffering from other health problems, making treatment and recovery more difficult.

Some diagnostic tests are less accurate in women, and many medications used to treat heart disease have not been tested in women, so their effectiveness is questionable. Additionally, treatment methods are not recommended to women as early in the disease process or as often, and this delay can result in poorer outcomes.[2, 3]

Women share some responsibility in creating this problem. We tend to delay seeking evaluation of chest pain. Although the first reaction to chest pain is denial that it may be a heart attack, diagnosis is further complicated by the fact that women do not associate the symptoms they are experiencing with their hearts. Unless they suffer the characteristic radiating left-side chest and arm pain that often is described as feeling like "an elephant sitting on my chest," they may attribute their symptoms to some other cause.

The other signs and symptoms of a heart attack that women need to be aware of include vague abdominal discomfort, nausea, vomiting, shortness of breath, upper back pain, fatigue, anxiety, and pallor. When a woman realizes that she is having difficulty, especially when the symptoms are not blatantly obvious, she may put off going to the doctor because she "does not have time." Women are so focused on the needs of others that their own needs often take a back seat. All of these factors prohibit the early detection of heart disease and can have a profound impact on the type of treatment received.

As a woman ages, her risk of heart disease increases as her estrogen levels decrease. For a sudden menopausal woman, who may sustain lower estrogen levels earlier in life, the risk for heart disease is even greater. However, as she struggles to cope with her menopausal symptoms and with the condition or disorder that brought on the sudden menopause, she may remain unaware of the long-term effects of estrogen loss. This is why it is important to work with your physician and educate yourself to address all of your health issues.

An Ounce of Prevention

Yes, the old adage holds true when it comes to heart disease: an ounce of prevention is definitely worth a pound of cure. In light of this, we can examine each risk factor and determine how taking the right steps can help prevent heart disease.

Smoking

There is absolutely nothing beneficial or glamorous about smoking. However, all you have to do is pick up a few magazines that appeal to young women, and you will find very glitzy advertisements for cigarettes. You can almost be fooled into thinking that smoking actually is healthy! Yet we know that just the opposite is true.

Women who smoke are two to six times more likely to have a heart attack than nonsmokers, and their risk for stroke also is higher. And a woman who smokes is less inclined to quit than a man who smokes.[4] The bottom line is that if you do not smoke, do not start. If you do smoke, quit.

Hypertension

High blood pressure is called the "silent killer" because there usually are no obvious symptoms in its early stages. For that reason, periodic blood pressure measurements are important. Blood pressure is the force of the blood against the walls of the arteries. It is expressed as a fraction. The systolic pressure, the top or first number, represents the force exerted on the arterial walls when the heart contracts. The diastolic pressure, the bottom or second number, is the force exerted on the arterial walls when the heart is between beats. A sustained blood pressure of 140/90 or greater is considered high.

Hypertension is a major risk factor for heart disease and stroke. The incidence is higher in African Americans and in postmenopausal women.

High Cholesterol

Cholesterol is a waxy substance produced by the body that is necessary for the body to function normally. Although the body produces all of the cholesterol it needs, we also get dietary cholesterol from foods of animal origin, such as meats and dairy products. In addition, dietary fat is derived from foods of animal origin and from some plant sources, such as nuts, seeds, and oils. Chapter 7 provides more detailed information on the various types of dietary fat, particularly the heart-healthy ones.

High levels of dietary cholesterol and, especially, high levels of certain kinds of fat in the diet can raise the levels of cholesterol circulating in the blood. High levels of blood cholesterol, in turn, can contribute to atherosclerosis, or abnormally high fatty deposits lining the arteries. This condition can lead to coronary artery disease. It is recommended that you keep your total blood cholesterol level lower than 200 mg/dl (milligrams per deciliter). A level of 200 to 239 mg/dl is considered borderline, and 240 mg/dl or greater is high.

However, your total cholesterol level isn't the whole story. Two other values that are important to monitor are high-density lipoproteins (HDL) and low-density lipoproteins (LDL). HDL is often referred to as the "good" cholesterol, because it carries cholesterol out of the arteries to the liver, where it is metabolized. By the same token, LDL is referred to as the "bad" cholesterol, because it carries cholesterol to the arteries. To protect the heart, HDL levels should be higher than 35 mg/dl (preferably around 60 mg/dl), and LDL levels should be lower than 130 mg/dl. It is interesting to note that one way in which estrogen appears to reduce a woman's risk of heart disease is by raising her HDL level and lowering her LDL level. Therefore, premenopausal women or postmenopausal women on estrogen may possess the ability to sustain a slightly higher total cholesterol level without an increased risk of heart disease.

Cholesterol levels are very dependent upon dietary fat and cholesterol. Therefore, keep your daily fat intake to less than 30 percent of your total calories (for the average woman, this works out to about 44 grams), saturated fat to less than 10 percent of total calories, and daily cholesterol intake to less than 300 mg.

To assess the average amount of fat in your diet, keep a 3-day food log. Be sure to record everything you eat and the amounts. After 3 days, consult a nutrient guide and read package labels to tally up the number of fat grams you have eaten. If you consume 2,000 calories a day, you can consume up to 44 grams of fat a day to obtain approximately 20 percent of your calories from fat. For the same 2,000-calorie diet, no more than 22 grams of saturated fat should be eaten. Since these numbers, including the number of calories you should ingest daily, vary based on individual factors, consult a registered dietitian to calculate your personal guidelines.

Occasionally, medications are needed to manage cholesterol levels.

Triglycerides

Triglycerides are a type of fatty substance manufactured by the body. When excess calories, dietary fat, or alcohol are ingested, triglyceride levels increase. In some studies, high levels of triglycerides have been linked to heart attacks in women.

According to the American Heart Association, blood triglyceride levels should remain below 200 mg/dl, and preferably below 150. As with cholesterol levels, you can reduce triglycerides by eating a low-fat diet, reducing weight, and increasing exercise. Eating 25 to 35 grams of fiber every day helps, too. As with cholesterol levels, medications are sometimes needed to manage triglyceride levels.

Obesity

It is estimated that 70 percent of women with coronary artery disease are overweight. People who are obese (more than 30 percent above their ideal body weight) are more likely to develop heart disease and stroke, even if no other risk factors are present.[5] The Framingham Heart Study found that the more overweight a women is, the higher her risk of heart disease.[6] According to the Harvard Nurses' Health Study, heart-attack risk is increased by 30 percent by being only 10 percent above ideal body weight.[7] Overweight women also are more likely to have low HDL levels, high triglyceride levels, hypertension, and diabetes.

Not only is percentage of body fat an indicator of heart disease; so is the distribution of that fat. Women with "apple-shaped" bodies, that is, who carry extra fat around the torso, have a higher risk of coronary artery disease than women with heavy hips and thighs, or "pear-shaped" women.

Sedentary Lifestyle

More studies are revealing what common sense has already told us. We need to get moving. Physical inactivity is an easily remedied risk factor for heart disease. It also influences other risk factors, such as blood pressure, cholesterol, triglycerides, and obesity.

To ensure long-term success, choose activities that you enjoy and are capable of doing, and set small, manageable goals. To reap optimal benefits, engage in physical activity for at least 30 minutes five to six times per week. Consider alternating aerobic activities—such as walking, dancing, swimming, tennis, and cycling—with an appropriate weight-training program. Aerobic exercise burns fat, and weight training builds muscle, which increases metabolism. It also is beneficial to increase your daily activity level by taking a few flights of stairs rather then taking the elevator, walking places instead of driving, and getting up out of the chair to retrieve items instead of asking others to get them for you.

Diabetes

Diabetes mellitus is the inability of the body to produce or respond to insulin properly. This leads to excessive amounts of glucose (sugar) in the blood and not enough in the cells. If untreated or uncontrolled, diabetes can precipitate kidney disease, blindness, and heart disease. Approximately 80 percent of all people with diabetes die of heart or blood-vessel disease.[8]

The most common form of diabetes is called type 2. It usually develops in adulthood and is typically non-insulin-dependent. (Type-1 diabetes, or insulin-dependent, is an autoimmune disease, whereby the body destroys the cells in the pancreas that manufacture insulin.) Type-2 diabetes is typically associated with lifestyle—specifically, with obesity and with diets high in sugar and other refined carbohydrates. The National Institutes of Health reports that 85 percent of all non-insulin-dependent diabetics are at least 20 percent overweight.[9] By the same token, type-2 diabetes is very responsive to weight loss and exercise, and in many cases can be controlled by lifestyle modification rather than oral medications.

Stress

The role played by stress in the development of heart disease has not been clearly defined by research. However, it is recognized that sustained levels of stress and the inability to effectively deal with that stress can lead to physical and emotional discord. In fact, studies have shown that emotions such as chronic anger and hostility increase the risk of hypertension, heart attack, and stroke.

When confronted with a stressful situation, whether real or perceived, the body responds by increasing the production of adrenaline and cortisol. This results in an increase in the vital signs (pulse, respiration, and blood pressure) and metabolism. In the case of intractable stress, our vital signs do not have a chance to lower. If blood pressure remains high, the arterial walls can be damaged.

Additionally, people who fail to manage stress effectively are more likely to partake in unhealthy behaviors, such as overeating, smoking, and drinking. Therefore, it is crucial that everyone identify her or his stressors and develop a plan to reduce them or find suitable outlets for dealing with them.

Depression

Evidence is mounting that depression increases the risk of heart attack. For years it has been known that depression following a heart attack decreased survival rates. Now there is strong evidence suggesting that a history of major depressive illness is a risk factor for heart attack. As noted earlier, chronic anger and hostility affect the heart in the same adverse manner, so it is very important that mood disorders be treated appropriately.

In her book *Her Healthy Heart,* Linda Ojeda also cites research further demonstrting the powerful impression that emotions make on a woman's heart. In addition to depression, stress, anger, and hostility, she discusses the detrimental effects of social isolation, loss of control, and emotional heartbreak.

Menopause

After menopause, a woman's risk of heart attack steadily rises. In the case of a sudden menopause, this risk rises sharply and quickly rather than gradually, and often years or decades earlier than with natural menopause. This is especially true for women who have undergone an early hysterectomy with BSO.

JUNE, a 57-year-old wife and mother, attended one of my Women and Heart Disease classes, during which we discussed the cardio-protective role of estrogen. After the class, June told me that she had her uterus and ovaries removed when she was 36 because of "female problems." She said that none of her doctors or nurses had even mentioned that she was at a higher risk of heart disease due to the surgery. She opted to discontinue estrogen replacement therapy after a few years because of a strong family history of breast cancer. Because she was "rarely ill," she did not visit her doctor regularly. As a result, June was very lax when it came to obtaining regular health screenings. Therefore, she had no idea what her blood pressure was or what her cholesterol and triglyceride levels were. Her heart health had never been a concern to her.

For June, attending my class was an important first step in understanding the relationship between sudden menopause and heart health. I then registered her for Heart Check, which is a screening program that assesses blood pressure, cholesterol, height and weight, and body fat composition. The results guided us in developing her health plan.

As stated earlier, estrogen has a cardioprotective effect through its ability to raise HDL and lower LDL cholesterol levels. Estrogen also benefits many women by lowering blood pressure and levels of fibrinogen, a blood-clotting component that is a predictor of stroke and heart attack. However, the results of the 1998 Heart and Estrogen/Progestin Replacement Study (HERS) demonstrated that women with established, advanced heart disease had a 50 percent increase in the risk of heart attack during the first year of estrogen use. Thereafter, their risk declined to that of women taking a placebo.[10]

In light of this study, it is imperative that the heart health of a sudden menopausal woman be assessed before she is placed on hormone replacement therapy. Keep in mind, though, that the results of this study pertained to women with advanced heart disease who had not undergone hysterectomies and who were placed on both estrogen and progestin.

Another study reported by the American Heart Association points to the role of prostaglandin, a hormone secreted by the uterus, in protecting women from heart disease.[11] If this is true, it is another hurdle to overcome for a woman who has had her uterus removed. Still, despite the hormonal changes that place sudden menopausal women at risk for heart disease, we are not defenseless. We have several powerful weapons in our cardioprotective arsenal. Never underestimate the impact that diet and exercise play in eliminating heart disease.

Heredity

If you have family members with coronary artery disease, you are more likely to develop it yourself. However, before resigning yourself to eventually developing heart disease, ask yourself this question: "Why are my relatives at risk?" If they are at risk because they eat a high-fat, low-fiber diet, smoke, and fail to exercise regularly, your hereditary risk might not be as high as you think. In other words, is the risk a matter primarily of genetics or of lifestyle?

On the other hand, do not assume that you are completely off the hook if heart disease does not run in your family. All it takes is an unhealthy lifestyle to catapult you into the high-risk category. Also, keep in mind that African Americans are at greater risk for heart disease. This is due, in part, to a higher incidence of hypertension.

Age

The relationship between age and heart disease is fairly simple: the older you get, the more likely you are to develop heart disease. However, leading a healthy lifestyle can substantially minimize the development of heart disease at any age.

To "B" or Not to "B"

When it comes to preventing and managing heart disease, the B vitamins are worth a look. Evidence is mounting that a diet low in folic acid, B-6 (pyridoxine), and B-12 (cyanocobalamin) may contribute toward coronary artery disease. It does this by allowing the amino acid homocysteine to accumulate in the blood, which leads to atherosclerosis.

Although a few large-scale studies have shown a predictive link between low levels of these B vitamins and cardiovascular disease, more evidence is needed before a definitive recommendation can be made about the effectiveness of increasing consumption of these vitamins in lowering heart disease. However, it appears that megadoses of folic acid, B-6, and B-12 are not needed to lower homocysteine levels. Simply obtaining the dietary reference intake (DRI) via diet or a multivitamin is adequate. This approach is both safe and prudent until further studies are conducted.[12]

Whether you are using B vitamins for your heart or for other reasons, keep in mind that the B vitamins work as a team, so it is best to take a B-complex supplement instead of a few of them individually. If you are taking a B complex to protect against the effects of stress or to improve mood and cognition, the higher doses that are recommended will help take care of your heart as well. (Chapter 5 includes additional information on vitamins.)

What About E?

Studies also are being performed on vitamin E and its link to heart disease. Thus far, vitamin E seems to offer a lot of cardioprotective potential. It is believed to reduce the risk of cardiovascular disease by preventing the oxidation of LDL (bad) cholesterol, thereby decreasing the likelihood of plaque formation within the arteries; by reducing the blood's ability to clot; and by stimulating the anti-inflammatory response within the blood vessels. Recommendations on vitamin E supplements are mostly based upon its reputation as an antioxidant and generally fall within the range of 400 to 800 IUs daily.

Coenzyme Q10 (CoQ10)

Also known as ubiquinone, coenzyme Q10 is found in small amounts in most foods. As a supplement, it has the most demonstrable effects on the heart. It enhances the utilization of oxygen, especially within the heart muscle. Not only can it be used preventively, but it can also facilitate cardiac functioning in patients with significant coronary artery disease, as well as those with congestive heart failure. A safe, therapeutic dosage for healthy adults is 60 to 100 mg per day.

Garlic

Garlic functions on several levels to guard against heart disease. It has the ability to reduce cholesterol, blood pressure, and blood clotting. And if that is not enough, garlic works as an anti-infective agent against bacteria and viruses. Garlic works best when eaten raw. The easiest way to go about incorporating garlic into your diet is to mince it and mix it with your food. Cooking it thoroughly can destroy some of the active ingredients.

If you cannot tolerate garlic raw, briefly sautéing it in a small amount of olive oil or broth, or softening it the same way in the microwave, is better than overcooking it. Cooking with garlic as often as possible is the most beneficial, but be sure to keep fresh parsley or a breath mint handy!

Some people use garlic supplements as an alternative, but they may not be as effective as fresh garlic. Most sources recommend taking the equivalent of one clove of garlic daily.

On the Horizon: Designer Estrogens

As mentioned in the chapter on osteoporosis, selective estrogen receptor modulators (SERMs), the so-called designer estrogens, mimic the effects of estrogen on the heart by reducing total cholesterol and LDL levels. Their attraction is that they do not stimulate breast tissue the way estrogen does; therefore, they offer another alternative to postmenopausal women who are not candidates for hormones or who do not wish to use hormones.

A Final Note

As you can see, we have power over many of the risk factors for heart disease. Even though estrogen plays a very influential role in maintaining heart health, lifestyle choices play an equally, if not more, important role. This is where our greatest potential exists in the battle against this disease. Heart disease is largely preventable and within the scope of our control. However, to reap the ultimate rewards, we must lay the foundation of healthy behaviors for our children and grandchildren. In this way, the vicious cycle of heart disease can be broken.

Chapter Highlights

- A sudden menopausal woman's risk of heart disease rises sharply as her hormone levels plummet. This is due to her body's greatly diminished levels of the cardioprotective hormone estrogen. The younger a woman is when sudden menopause occurs, the longer the heart remains without the benefits of estrogen.

- Due to this hormonal deprivation, it is especially important for a sudden menopausal woman to adopt a healthy lifestyle and stick to it. In this way, she can nullify many deleterious effects on heart health caused by the loss of estrogen.

- You can learn how to lead a heart-healthy lifestyle. Some of the changes you may need to incorporate into your life include: eating a low-fat, high-fiber diet; exercising daily; quitting smoking; maintaining a healthy weight; practicing relaxation techniques; and seeking help for mood disorders.

 If you like garlic, use it at least three times a week in your cooking. After consulting a qualified herbalist or naturopath, consider supplementing your diet with vitamin B complex, vitamin E, and coenzyme Q10. If you are taking any medication, be sure to check with your doctor or pharmacist regarding possible interactions.

Doc Talk

 Evaluate your risk factors for heart disease with your doctor. Discuss ways of lowering your risk.

 Work with your doctor to devise a health-screening schedule. Cardiac screening tests include total cholesterol, HDL cholesterol, LDL cholesterol, triglycerides, blood sugar, and blood pressure. Be sure to determine the frequency of these screenings so you will know how often to have them done (see Chapter 7 for guidelines). Depending on your personal and family history of heart disease, as well as the results of your screening tests, you may require other diagnostic testing.

 Talk to your doctor about medication options available (HRT, SERMs, aspirin) to lower your risk of heart disease, and ask if you are a candidate for any of these approaches.

 If you think you will need help in breaking unhealthy habits, ask for referrals to the appropriate professionals and programs. Assistance may come in the form of nutrition counseling, weight-loss groups, smoking-cessation programs, exercise classes, cooking classes, and stress-management programs.

5

Making It Through the Maze of Dietary Supplements

While performing a nutritional assessment on *CARRIE*, a 38-year-old aide in a group home, I asked her to list any vitamins and herbs she was using. Fortunately, she brought the bottles with her, because there were so many I was having difficulty keeping them straight. After totaling the doses of the various supplements, I realized she was overdosing on some and underdosing on others. When I asked her why she was taking the various products, she replied, "I just wanted to feel better, so I asked several of my friends what they were taking and bought those. I suppose that wasn't very wise." After determining her goals for using supplements, I helped her streamline her vitamin regimen.

Using This Chapter

In Chapter 2, I identified various coping strategies for some of the changes that can accompany a sudden menopause. Included in those lists were dietary supplements that may be helpful in alleviating menopausal discomforts and annoyances. However, before you run out and buy them by the cartload, you need to become knowledgeable about vitamins, minerals, and herbs. This chapter is designed to provide a foundation from which to build your knowledge base about nutritional supplements.

It is essential that these products be used responsibly. This means being adequately informed about what you are taking. It is important to gather information about origin, dosage, duration of use, side effects, drug interactions, and synergistic relationships with other substances. A certified herbalist or knowledgeable pharmacist or nutritionist can tell you if there exist any interactions among foods, supplements, and medications of which you should be aware. As a general rule of thumb, allow at least 2 hours to elapse between taking medication and taking nutritional supplements. Some people mistakenly believe that because no prescription is required to buy these preparations, they can be used indiscriminately. This line of thinking can be dangerous. It also is inadvisable to discontinue taking prescribed medication without talking to your doctor—not only a certified herbalist. Just because you wish to embrace a more naturalistic approach to your health does not mean you should totally disregard Western medicine and technology. The premise of complementary medicine is that it integrates the principles of allopathy (conventional Western medicine) and naturopathy (traditional medicine). They are not mutually exclusive; they can coexist.

Dietary supplements may be a good alternative for the sudden menopausal woman who is not a candidate for or who does not wish to use hormone therapy. Appropriate use of supplements can help alleviate sudden menopausal changes such as hot flashes, night sweats, and cognitive changes.

Important notes:

1. If you are currently receiving chemotherapy or radiation for cancer, do not use any dietary supplements that function as antioxidants without consulting your oncologist. Many health authorities discourage use of antioxidants during treatment for cancer, because antioxidants may counteract the effects of chemotherapy and radiation on the tumor.

2. It is crucial that, for at least two weeks prior to any invasive procedure or surgery, you stop taking any supplements that

prolong bleeding time. Discuss this with your doctor before scheduling the test or operation.

3. Meet with the anesthesiologist prior to any procedure or surgery that requires anesthesia, and inform him/her of any vitamins or herbs you may be taking. Some herbs interact with anesthesia, and it can be dangerous to combine the two.

As *EMILY*, a 51-year-old clerk, put it, "I use different vitamins to help control my symptoms, but I still take the medicine my doctor prescribed. This way I get the best of both worlds." Because Emily took the time and effort to become informed about the supplements she was taking, she was able to use a very low dosage of estrogen in conjunction with vitamins and soy products. This combined therapy helped her to achieve control over her hot flashes, vaginal dryness, and cognitive impairment.

Vitamins and Minerals

Vitamins and minerals are essential to life. The numerous functions they fuel include the formation of blood cells, production of hormones, regulation of the nervous system, and maintenance of cell and tissue integrity. Most vitamins and minerals are not produced in the body or are done so in insufficient quantities. They are referred to as micronutrients, because the amounts required for normal functioning are miniscule. However, a slight deficiency in even one vitamin may result in bodily disharmony.

Macronutrients are substances that provide us with energy (for example, carbohydrates, protein, fat) and are consumed in greater quantities. However, without micronutrients, macronutrients could not be digested and used as energy.

Another way of looking at it is to think of vitamins as coenzymes. They need the enzymes in food in order to work. This is the reason that vitamins cannot be used as a substitute for a nutritious diet. In addition, food is a source of protein, fiber, phytochemicals (vital substances from plant sources), and energy. If you skip meals or just eat junk food, popping a vitamin pill will not help.

Vitamins are categorized as fat-soluble or water-soluble. Fat-soluble vitamins (vitamins A, D, E, and K) require an adequate supply of fat to be absorbed. Since they are stored in the liver, extended use of megadoses of these vitamins can be toxic.

Water-soluble vitamins (the B vitamins and vitamin C) do not require fat for absorption. They need to be replenished daily because excess amounts are simply excreted in the urine. However, prolonged usage of megadoses of these vitamins also can be harmful.

When fat-soluble and water-soluble vitamins are used in responsible dosages, side effects are rare. Nevertheless, if you are on medication, check with a pharmacist or dietitian to determine if you should be aware of any drug-nutrient interactions. For example, many antioxidants and herbs can prolong bleeding time, which could be detrimental to women taking anticoagulants (blood thinners). Conversely, vitamin K, which acts as a coagulant, can inhibit the effects of certain prescription blood thinners.

Minerals are elements in the body that are just as important as vitamins. They are vital for bone structure, muscle contraction, blood formation, heartbeat, fluid balance, and nerve impulses. They are categorized as either essential minerals or trace minerals.

Calcium, sodium, and potassium are examples of essential minerals. They are required by the body in larger amounts than trace minerals.

Although smaller amounts of trace minerals are needed, this should not discount their importance. Examples of trace minerals include iron, zinc, and fluoride.

Considering the crucial need for vitamins and minerals in the body, how do we know the right amounts to ingest? The Food and Nutrition Board, part of the National Research Council of the National Academy of Sciences, devised the Recommended Daily Allowances (RDAs) for vitamins and minerals. The RDAs serve as an estimate of the amounts needed for normal growth in children and to prevent nutritional deficiencies in adults. Many scientists and nutrition experts believe that the RDA levels are very inadequate and do not reflect the latest research on vitamins and their potential to prevent diseases. That is why, for easing menopausal changes, some sources list therapeutic ranges of vitamins that vastly exceed the RDAs.

According to this philosophy, the RDA would not be considered an optimal intake. However, in the past few years, the Food and Nutrition Board has recognized the inadequacy of the RDAs and has developed a different reference system. The new term is dietary reference intake (DRI).

DRI is a generic term that refers to several reference values, including RDAs and tolerable upper intake levels (UL). However, DRIs and tolerable upper intake levels have not yet been established for all of the vitamins and minerals. In this chapter, I will provide them when available; otherwise, I will list the RDAs.

Important note: The "common dosages" listed below are simply typical dosages that many postmenopausal women use. Most of this information comes from the experience of naturopathic practitioners or clinicians schooled in nutritional supplements. These dosages are not established or endorsed by any governing agency or clinical organization. Sometimes, therefore, these dosages exceed the tolerable upper intake level, which is defined as the "maximum level of daily nutrient intake that is unlikely to cause side effects in nearly all of the individuals for whom it is recommended." Often, however, the "common dosages" fall in the same range as the RDA or DRI for a given nutrient.

Although the "common dosages" are not unusual, individual responses to these substances do vary. It is best to take the lowest amount of a supplement that will diminish your menopausal symptoms and then monitor yourself for side effects. If side effects do occur, stop taking the supplement. If the side effects are minor, you may wish to reintroduce the vitamin at a much lower dosage. It also is beneficial if you can locate a knowledgeable health professional or a certified natural health professional to help get you started.

Many RDAs and DRIs are considered too low to exert a therapeutic effect. But keep in mind that RDA guidelines originated
from a need to prevent diseases that result from a long-term deficiency of vitamins. For example, scurvy, which is caused by a deficiency in vitamin C and is practically unheard of in the United
States today, was rampant among sailors who consumed a diet
lacking in fruits and vegetables while confined to ships on the high
seas. Signs and symptoms of scurvy included bleeding gums, tooth
loss, pain in the limbs and joints, and weakness. Scurvy was the
cause of many deaths until the origin of the disease was determined and fruit was added to the diet.

A serious condition such as scurvy should not be confused
with a marginal deficiency. A marginal nutritional deficiency is a
condition in which the body's vitamin and mineral stores are gradually and progressively depleted, resulting in the loss of optimal
health and the impairment of bodily processes. Initially, such a
condition goes undetected. If uncorrected, physical and emotional
changes occur.

A marginal loss is one stop along the deficiency continuum. If
allowed to continue, it can develop into a deficiency disease.[1] For
this reason, experts who are proactive about the use of dietary
supplements generally recommend dosages higher than the DRI.
This holds true for relief of symptoms associated with sudden
menopause.

Getting Started

DAWN, a 42-year-old teacher, wanted to know how to alleviate
the sudden menopausal symptoms that commenced after her hysterectomy with BSO. When I began our session by performing a
lifestyle assessment—which included an analysis of her diet—she
said, "No, you don't understand. I'd like to try natural remedies,
but I don't know where to start." She was very surprised that I was
spending time giving her pointers on her diet and didn't immediately jump into discussing vitamins and herbs.

Often, people read about a particular nutrient, decide they need it, and begin taking it without first evaluating their diet. This is the equivalent of applying a Band-Aid to a gaping wound. It is not going to be of much help. However, you can feel significantly better by making the correct dietary changes.

I will be addressing lifestyle modification in more detail in Chapter 7, but for now, it would be helpful for you to keep a daily eating record for at least 3 days (one of which should be a weekend day). Then compare your diet to the recommendations outlined in the Food Guide Pyramid, or show it to a dietitian. This will help you determine if you need to increase the number of servings of a particular type of food. If this is the case, I recommend beginning there before adding various dietary supplements.

Once you decide to supplement your diet, begin with a multivitamin. Vitamins and minerals function interdependently. One works best when the others are present. If some are missing, it may cause a greater imbalance. A multivitamin will provide you with broad-spectrum coverage of most vitamins and possibly some minerals as well.

This type of synergistic relationship is present with the B vitamins; with calcium, magnesium, phosphorous, and vitamin D; and with iron and vitamin C, to name a few. Additional amounts of an individual vitamin or mineral—such as calcium or vitamin C—can be taken if the multivitamin does not contain the required amount or if a larger amount is needed to alleviate a particular symptom—such as hot flashes or mood swings.

After you have decided upon the supplements you wish to try, the next hurdle to clear is buying them. It can be quite overwhelming to stand in front of countless shelves full of dietary aids trying to decide which one to buy.

The first decision to make is whether to buy a brand name or a generic product. This is a debatable issue further complicated by the fact that many brand-name companies manufacture vitamins for store brands. If you are considering a chain-store brand and the chain has an in-store pharmacist, ask the pharmacist if another company sells its vitamins under the store label. In most instances, you are getting the exact same product at a lower cost.

It also is a good idea to compare the labels between brand names and off-brand names. Many contain the same ingredients in the same or comparable amounts. You may want to consult a naturopathic practitioner for some recommendations regarding reputable brands of supplements. Some of my favorite brands include Nature's Sunshine, Biotics, Twin Lab, Natrol, Enzymatic Therapy, Solgar, Standard Process, Inc., and Herbalist and Alchemist.

The second hurdle to overcome is whether to buy a natural or a synthetic version of a product. This issue continues to be controversial. Proponents of natural products claim this form is essential because there may be substances derived from plants that are needed to utilize the vitamins. On the flip side are those who favor synthetic products because, they say, the substances are chemically similar to what the body produces naturally and are utilized the same way in our bodies. Synthetic products also tend to be less expensive. To me, of greater importance than deciding on a natural or synthetic product is to be sure whatever product you choose is as free of as many fillers and additives as possible.

Despite the debate, there does seem to be a consensus regarding vitamin E. Natural vitamin E (d-alpha tocopherol or mixed-d tocopherols) seems to be absorbed better than the synthetic version (dl-alpha tocopherol).[2] Experts also recommend using the organic form of selenium. Other than vitamin E and selenium, I tell my clients that either form is acceptable.

Before taking your purchases to the checkout counter, take a few moments to make some observations. Does your selection have an expiration date on it? Is the product still good? If your choices do not contain expiration dates, put them back. Vitamins and minerals lose their potency over time. Also, the products you choose should have some type of safety seal to prevent tampering, and they should be stored in a cool, dry location.

When the vitamins finally make it home with you, make the most of the time and money you have invested by remembering to take them. Establish some type of routine so taking them becomes second nature. As a general rule, don't take your vitamins on an empty stomach. Food will enhance absorption and minimize the gastric upset reported by some people when taking vitamins.

If you bought a multivitamin and individual vitamins, begin taking the multivitamin first. After a week, add one other vitamin. Gradually add the remaining vitamins at 1-week intervals. This way, if an intolerance or an allergic reaction occurs, it will be easier to determine which product is the culprit.

You now need to adjust the dosage of some of the supplements on a daily basis, depending on your daily need. For example, if on a particular day you have consumed foods rich in calcium, then you may want to decrease your calcium supplement accordingly.

If this approach is unappealing to you, another option would be to check your 3-day food diary and, by consulting a nutrition book, determine the amount of calcium you are eating. Add up the amount of calcium you are getting every day, and take an average for the 3 days. Subtract this number from the amount you need every day (between 1,200 mg and 1,500 mg), and that will tell you how much calcium you need to supplement on a daily basis.

This also may be the case with vitamin C. Many people calculate their ascorbic acid (vitamin C) intake not only by their daily consumption of fruits and vegetables, but by the amount of stress or illness they are experiencing. During times of high stress or illness, you may choose to increase your vitamin C intake.

If you are taking vitamin C supplements, divide them up over the course of the day rather than taking the day's dosage all at once. Multiple divided doses of 250 mg to 500 mg make the ascorbic acid more available to your body all day long. Time-released vitamin C is another alternative.

Since your requirements for vitamins change over the years, you may need to fine-tune your regimen depending on your needs. Keep in mind that dietary supplements work gradually. It may take a few months before you realize the maximum benefits.

One last note before you consult the following list of vitamins and minerals: swallow your vitamins with an 8-ounce glass of water. This increases the bioavailability of the vitamins.

Recall the dissolution test from Chapter 3. To test whether your vitamins are capable of being absorbed by your body, perform this test: place the vitamin in ½ cup of white vinegar for ½ hour, stirring every 5 minutes. After 30 minutes have elapsed, the vitamin should have dissolved or at least be partially disintegrated. Many vitamin manufacturers are now listing adherence to dissolution testing on their product labels.

Dietary Supplements: A to Zinc

The amounts recommended are suitable for adult females.

Important note: Nutrient-nutrient and nutrient-medication interactions can occur. If you are taking medication, before beginning to take supplements please check with a dietitian or pharmacist for possible side effects and contraindications. Otherwise, consulting a qualified herbalist, naturopath, or health professional for guidance is recommended.

Water-Soluble Vitamins

Note: Although I have listed the various B vitamins separately, it is best to take them as a B complex. Be sure to get the entire complement of B vitamins in your supplement. Most women do well with a B-100-B-complex tablet.

Thiamin (B-1)

DRI: 25–50 years of age—1.1 mg
  51+ years of age—1.1 mg

Common dosage (not established or endorsed by any governmental or scientific agency; see discussion above, under heading "Vitamins and Minerals"): 50 mg to 100 mg

Functions: metabolism; functioning of nervous system, heart, and muscles; works synergistically with other B vitamins

Food sources: whole grains, fortified breads and cereals, lean meats, pork, fish, dried beans, soybeans, peanuts, brewer's yeast, garbanzo beans, kidney beans, peas

>peas, boiled, ½ cup—.21 mg
>
>lean ham, 3½ oz.—.75 mg
>
>skim milk, 1 cup—.09 mg
>
>Wheaties, 1 cup—.37 mg
>
>brown rice, 1 cup—.20 mg
>
>raisins, seedless, ⅔ cup—.16 mg
>
>pineapple, canned, 1 cup—.24 mg
>
>brewer's yeast, 1 oz.—4.43 mg

Adverse reactions: rare; may include nausea, diarrhea, restlessness, skin rash, itching

Riboflavin (B-2)

DRI: 25–50 years of age—1.1 mg
  51+ years of age—1.1 mg

Common dosage (not established or endorsed by any governmental or scientific agency; see discussion above, under heading "Vitamins and Minerals"): 50 mg to 100 mg

Functions: metabolism; functioning of nervous system, eyes, and skin; production of red blood cells; works synergistically with other B vitamins

Food sources: milk, dairy products, fortified breads and cereals, lean meats, eggs, legumes, green leafy vegetables, nuts

>skim milk, 1 cup—.34 mg
>
>1 egg—.26 mg
>
>kidney beans, ½ cup—.12 mg
>
>spinach, boiled, ½ cup—.21 mg
>
>skinless chicken breast, ½—.10 mg
>
>Frosted Mini Wheats, 4 pieces—.43 mg

Adverse reactions: rare; may include nausea, vomiting

Niacin (B-3)

DRI: 25–50 years of age—14 mg
51+ years of age—14 mg

Common dosage (not established or endorsed by any governmental or scientific agency; see discussion above, under heading "Vitamins and Minerals"): 50 mg to 100 mg

Tolerable upper intake level: 35 mg

Functions: metabolism; functioning of nervous system, skin, and digestive tract; reduces cholesterol and triglycerides; works synergistically with other B vitamins

Food sources: fortified breads and cereals, dairy products, lean meats, fish, eggs, nuts
   skinless chicken breast, ½—11.8 mg
   salmon, 3 oz.—8.6 mg
   Raisin Bran, ¾ cup—5.0 mg
   peanut butter, 2 tbsp.—4.2 mg
   ground beef, extra lean, broiled, 3½ oz.—5.0 mg
   brewer's yeast, 1 oz.—10.7 mg

Adverse reactions: noted in high doses; may include abdominal pain, nausea, vomiting, diarrhea, headache, feeling flushed, itching

Pyridoxine (B-6)

DRI: 25–50 years of age—1.3 mg
51+ years of age—1.5 mg

Common dosage (not established or endorsed by any governmental or scientific agency; see discussion above, under heading "Vitamins and Minerals"): 50 mg to 100 mg

Tolerable upper intake level: 100 mg

Functions: metabolism; needed for chemical reactions of proteins and amino acids; formation of neurotransmitters;

brain functioning; production of red blood cells; synthesizes
antibodies in the immune system; believed to protect against
heart disease by reducing homocysteine levels; works
synergistically with other B vitamins

Food sources: fortified breads and cereals, whole grains, lean
meats, fish, beans, legumes, nuts, bananas, avocados, rice,
carrots

> banana, 1 medium—.66 mg
>
> avocado, medium, ½—.43 mg
>
> canned tuna, in water, 3 oz.—.3 mg
>
> beef, top sirloin, 3½ oz.—.43 mg
>
> Grape Nut flakes, ⅞ cup—.50 mg
>
> potato, baked, with skin—.70 mg

Adverse reactions: rare; may include numbness or tingling of
extremities, drowsiness, clumsiness, unsteady gait

Folic Acid (Folate, B-9)

DRI: 25–50 years of age—400 mcg
51+ years of age—400 mcg

Common dosage (not established or endorsed by any
governmental or scientific agency; see discussion above,
under heading "Vitamins and Minerals"): 400 mcg

Tolerable upper intake level: 1,000 mcg

Functions: DNA synthesis; production of red blood cells;
reduces the risk of birth defects; possibly reduces the risk of
colon cancer; believed to protect against heart disease by
reducing homocysteine levels; works synergistically with
other B vitamins

Food sources: whole grains, rice, green leafy vegetables,
garbanzo beans, lentils, citrus fruits, brewer's yeast, broccoli,
asparagus, beets, sweet potatoes

> orange, 1 medium—47 mcg
>
> avocado, medium, ½—81 mcg

    garbanzo beans, ½ cup—80 mcg

    lentils, ½ cup—180 mcg

    spinach, boiled, ½ cup—131 mcg

    Corn Flakes, 1 cup—100 mcg

Adverse reactions: rare; may include diarrhea, skin rash, general malaise

Cobalamin (B-12)

DRI: 25–50 years of age—2.4 mcg
    51+ years of age—2.4 mcg

Common dosage (not established or endorsed by any governmental or scientific agency; see discussion above, under heading "Vitamins and Minerals"): 50 mcg to 100 mcg

Functions: metabolism; normal functioning of the nervous system; production of red blood cells; believed to protect against heart disease by reducing homocysteine levels; works synergistically with other B vitamins

Food sources: animal products (milk and milk products, eggs, poultry, meat, fish, organ meats) and fortified foods

    canned tuna, in water, 3 oz.—2.45 mcg

    skim milk, 1 cup—.93 mcg

    1 egg—.56 mcg

    skinless chicken, 3½ oz.—.34 mcg

    haddock, 3 oz.—1.02 mcg

    cottage cheese, low-fat, ½ cup—.71 mcg

    Cheerios, 1¼ cup—1.50 mcg

Adverse reactions: rare; may include diarrhea

Pantothenic Acid (B-5)

DRI: No deficiencies have been observed in humans, so no DRI exists. The estimated safe and adequate daily dietary intake is 5 mg.

Common dosage (not established or endorsed by any governmental or scientific agency; see discussion above, under heading "Vitamins and Minerals"): 50 mg to 100 mg

Functions: metabolism; synthesis of body chemicals (for example, cholesterol, hormones); formation of the neurotransmitter acetylcholine; works synergistically with other B vitamins

Food sources: whole-grain products, wheat germ, meats, eggs, fish, brewer's yeast, soybeans, peas, lentils, sunflower seeds

>skinless chicken, 3½ oz.—.97 mg
>
>skim milk, 1 cup—.81 mg
>
>oatmeal, cooked, 1 cup—.47 mg
>
>grapefruit, ½—.35 mg
>
>strawberries, 1 cup—.51 mg
>
>broccoli, boiled, ½ cup—.40 mg
>
>potato, baked, with skin—1.12 mg

Adverse reactions: rare; may include diarrhea

Biotin (B-7)

DRI: No deficiencies have been observed in humans, so no DRI exists. The estimated safe and adequate daily dietary intake is 30 mcg.

Common dosage (not established or endorsed by any governmental or scientific agency; see discussion above, under heading "Vitamins and Minerals"): 50 mcg to 100 mcg

Functions: metabolism; formation of fatty acids; protein synthesis; similar to pantothenic acid and B-12; works synergistically with other B vitamins

Food sources: whole grains, brewer's yeast, poultry, meat, fish, milk and milk products, brown rice, peas, lentils, oats, walnuts, cashews, sunflower seeds

>oatmeal, cooked, ½ cup—6.0 mcg
>
>1 egg—10.0 mcg

skim milk, 1 cup—10.0 mcg

macaroni and cheese, from mix, ¾ cup—3.0 mcg

brown rice, cooked, ½ cup—9.0 mcg

peanut butter, 2 tbsp.—12.0 mcg

salmon, 3 oz.—10.0 mcg

Adverse reactions: none expected

Ascorbic Acid (Vitamin C)

DRI: 25–50 years of age—75 mg
  51+ years of age—75 mg

Common dosage (not established or endorsed by any governmental or scientific agency; see discussion above, under heading "Vitamins and Minerals"): 500 mg to 1,000 mg

Tolerable upper intake level: 2,000 mg

Functions: antioxidant; healthy gums and teeth; collagen production; tissue/wound repair; iron absorption

Food sources: citrus fruits, strawberries, tomatoes, broccoli, collards, kale, potatoes, spinach, sweet and hot peppers

orange, 1 medium—80 mg

strawberries, 1 cup—85 mg

cantaloupe, 1 cup—68 mg

kiwi, 1 medium—75 mg

papaya, 1 medium—188 mg

broccoli, boiled, ½ cup—58 mg

yellow pepper, 1 medium—341 mg

grapefruit juice, frozen, 8 oz.—83 mg

orange juice, frozen, 8 oz.—97 mg

Adverse reactions: rare; may include indigestion, diarrhea, nausea, vomiting

Fat-Soluble Vitamins

Vitamin A/Beta-Carotene

(Beta-carotene is a pre-vitamin A compound found in plants. The body converts it to vitamin A. For use as an antioxidant, take beta-carotene or mixed carotenoids.)

RDA: 25–50 years of age—4,000 IU or 800 RE (Retinol Equivalents) of vitamin A
51+ years of age—4,000 IU or 800 RE of vitamin A

Common dosage (not established or endorsed by any governmental or scientific agency; see discussion above, under heading "Vitamins and Minerals"): 4,000 IU of vitamin A; 15,000 IU to 25,000 IU of beta-carotene or mixed carotenoids

Functions: antioxidant*; vision; healthy skin, teeth, mucous membranes, bones, and soft tissue

*studies using supplements have shown conflicting results. May be harmful if used by smokers

Food sources: carrots, broccoli, winter squash, pumpkin, sweet potatoes, apricots, watermelon, endive, kale, leaf lettuce

Note: Quantities listed below refer to the amount of vitamin A
carrot, raw, 1 medium—20,253 IU
sweet potato, boiled, without skin, ½ cup mashed—27,968 IU
winter squash, baked, ½ cup—3,628 IU
apricots, dried, 10 halves—2,534 IU
broccoli, boiled, ½ cup—1,082 IU
spinach, boiled, ½ cup—7,371 IU
cantaloupe, 1 cup—5,158 IU
mango, 1 medium—8,060 IU
liver, beef, braised, 3½ oz.—35,679 IU

Adverse reactions (vitamin A): may include appetite loss, abdominal pain, hair loss, headache, bone or joint pain, drying or cracking of skin or lips. High doses of beta-carotene may result in an orange-yellow tint to the skin

Calciferol (Vitamin D)

DRI: 25–50 years of age—200 IU (5 mcg)
   51–70 years of age—400 IU (10 mcg)
   71+ years of age—600 IU (15 mcg)

Common dosage (not established or endorsed by any governmental or scientific agency; see discussion above, under heading "Vitamins and Minerals"): 400 IU to 800 IU

Tolerable upper intake level: 1,000 IU

Functions: absorption of calcium; maintains proper blood levels of calcium and phosphorus; necessary for bone health; manufactured by the body after exposure to daylight or sunshine

Food sources: fortified milk, cheese, butter, margarine, fortified cereals, fish, egg yolks
   1 egg—25 IU
   fortified skim milk, 1 cup—100 IU
   salmon, 3½ oz.—150–550 IU
   shrimp, 3½ oz.—150 IU
   mackerel, 3½ oz.—1,100 IU
   sardines, canned, 3½ oz.—1,150–1,570 IU

Adverse reactions: may include nausea, vomiting, diarrhea, constipation, appetite loss, headache, dry mouth, metallic taste, mental confusion

Tocopherol (Vitamin E; d-alpha tocopherol or mixed-d tocopherols is the natural form.)

DRI: 25–50 years of age—22 IU
   51+ years of age—22 IU

Common dosage (not established or endorsed by any governmental or scientific agency; see discussion above, under heading "Vitamins and Minerals"): 400 IU to 800 IU

Tolerable upper intake level: 1,500 IU

Functions: antioxidant; formation of red blood cells; anticoagulant (studies are underway to determine if vitamin E reduces the risk of heart disease, Alzheimer's disease, cancer, and cataracts). Functions synergistically with selenium.

Food sources: vegetable oils, margarine, wheat germ, corn, nuts, sunflower seeds, olives, green leafy vegetables, asparagus, sweet potatoes

asparagus, 5 spears—1.1–1.6 IU

dried prunes, 10—1.61–1.85 IU

avocado, ½—.95–2.0 IU

spinach, ½ cup—2.2–3.3 IU

peaches, canned, ½ cup—2.1–2.4 IU

safflower oil, ¼ cup—19.5 IU

Adverse reactions: may include blurred vision, fatigue, nausea, abdominal pain, diarrhea, dizziness, headache

Minerals

Calcium

DRI: 25–50 years of age—1,000 mg
51+ years of age—1,200 mg

Note: The National Institutes of Health recommends 1,000 mg for postmenopausal women on hormones and 1,500 mg for postmenopausal women not on hormones as well as for all women over age 65.

Common dosage (not established or endorsed by any governmental or scientific agency; see discussion above, under heading "Vitamins and Minerals"): 1,200 mg to 1,500 mg

Tolerable upper intake level: 2,500 mg

Functions: builds strong bones and teeth; regulates heartbeat, muscle contractions, blood clotting; may improve PMS symptoms

Food sources: soy milk, cow's milk and milk products, broccoli, tempeh, tofu, canned sardines and salmon (with bones), macaroni and cheese, pizza, molasses, almonds, Brazil nuts, spinach, collard greens, figs, apricots, baked beans

    skim milk, 1 cup—302 mg

    cheddar cheese, low-fat, 1 oz.—200 mg

    plain yogurt, low-fat, 8 oz.—400 mg

    calcium-fortified orange juice, 1 cup—300 mg

    sardines, with bones, 3 oz.—371 mg

    Brazil nuts, 1 oz.—50 mg

    black-eyed peas, ½ cup—105 mg

    kale, ½ cup—90 mg

    collard greens, boiled, ½ cup—179 mg

    blackstrap molasses, 1 tbsp.—172 mg

    salmon, canned with bones, 3 oz.—181 mg

Adverse reactions: may include nausea, constipation, appetite loss, dry mouth

Phosphorus

DRI: 25–50 years of age—700 mg
    51+ years of age—700 mg

Common dosage (not established or endorsed by any governmental or scientific agency; see discussion above, under heading "Vitamins and Minerals"): 700 mg

Functions: energy production; builds strong bones and teeth; formation of genetic material

Food sources: meat, fish, poultry, dairy products, eggs, peas, beans, nuts

skim milk, 1 cup—247 mg

yogurt, low-fat, 8 oz.—250 mg

skinless chicken breast, roasted, ½—196 mg

kidney beans, ½ cup—120 mg

pumpkin seeds, roasted, 1 oz.—333 mg

sunflower seeds, dry-roasted, 1 oz.—328 mg

Life cereal, 1 oz.—162 mg

Adverse reactions: excess amounts can impair the body's use of iron, calcium, and magnesium

Magnesium

DRI: 25–30 years of age—310 mg
30–50 years of age—320 mg
51+ years of age—320 mg

Common dosage (not established or endorsed by any governmental or scientific agency; see discussion above, under heading "Vitamins and Minerals"): 300 mg to 400 mg

Tolerable upper intake level: 350 mg

Functions: bone growth; functioning of nerves, bones, and muscles; regulation of heartbeat

Food sources: whole grains, green leafy vegetables, meat, fish, milk, nuts, wheat germ, molasses, sunflower seeds, almonds

skim milk, 1 cup—28 mg

Swiss chard, boiled, ½ cup—76 mg

almonds, dry-roasted, 1 oz.—86 mg

garbanzo beans, ½ cup—35 mg

artichoke, boiled, 1 medium—72 mg

cashews, dry-roasted, 1 oz.—74 mg

halibut, 3 oz.—91 mg

sunflower seeds, dry-roasted, 1 oz.—37 mg

banana, 1 medium—33 mg

figs, dried, 5—56 mg

bran cereal, 1 oz.—122 mg

Adverse reactions: may include abdominal pain, nausea, vomiting, diarrhea, appetite loss, irregular heartbeat, mood changes, fatigue

Iron

RDA: 25–50 years of age—15 mg

51+ years of age—10 mg

Common dosage (not established or endorsed by any governmental or scientific agency; see discussion above, under heading "Vitamins and Minerals"): 10 mg to 15 mg

Functions: formation of hemoglobin (carries oxygen in the blood) and myoglobin (carries oxygen in muscle); part of enzymes and protein

Food sources: red meat, liver, poultry, fish, egg yolk, peas, beans, nuts, dried fruits, green leafy vegetables, fortified cereals, molasses, garbanzo beans, pumpkin, wheat germ

ground beef, extra lean, baked, 3½ oz.—2.96 mg

liver, beef, braised, 3½ oz.—6.77 mg

raisins, seedless, ⅔ cup—2.08 mg

1 egg—.6 mg

black beans, boiled, 1 cup—3.60 mg

spinach, boiled, ½ cup—3.21 mg

garbanzo beans, 1 cup—3.23 mg

lentils, boiled, 1 cup—6.59 mg

figs, dried, 5—2.09 mg

Cream of Wheat, quick, cooked, ¾ cup—7.6 mg

Adverse reactions: may include abdominal pain, black stools, diarrhea, vomiting

Selenium

DRI: 25–50 years of age—55 mcg
51+ years of age—55 mcg

Common dosage (not established or endorsed by any governmental or scientific agency; see discussion above, under heading "Vitamins and Minerals"): 200 mcg to 400 mcg

Tolerable upper intake level: 400 mcg

Functions: antioxidant; enhances immunity; preliminary research suggests it plays a role in preventing cancer and heart disease; works synergistically with vitamin E

Food sources: meat, seafood, whole grains
skinless chicken breast, ½—24 mcg
canned tuna, in water, 3 oz.—60 mcg
ground beef, lean, 3½ oz.—30 mcg
1 egg—16 mcg
whole wheat bread, 1 slice—9.5 mcg

Adverse reactions: may include nausea, diarrhea, irritability, numbness or tingling in extremities

Zinc

RDA: 25–50 years of age—12 mg
51+ years of age—12 mg

Common dosage (not established or endorsed by any governmental or scientific agency; see discussion above, under heading "Vitamins and Minerals"): 15 mg to 30 mg

Functions: growth and development; wound healing; DNA synthesis; maintains normal taste and smell; functioning of immune system

Food sources: seafood, turkey, meat, liver, egg yolk, whole-grain products, molasses, seeds, wheat germ, brewer's yeast, milk

> chuck roast, lean, braised, 3½ oz.—10.27 mg
>
> turkey, light meat without skin, roasted, 3½ oz.—2.04 mg
>
> sunflower seeds, dry-roasted, 1 oz.—1.50 mg
>
> Special K cereal, 1⅓ cup—3.75 mg

Adverse reactions: may include nausea, vomiting, diarrhea, abdominal pain, gastric ulceration

Other Supplements

Lecithin

DRI: No DRI exists. Lecithin is the primary source of choline. The adequate intake level of choline for adult females is 425 mg.

Common dosage (not established or endorsed by any governmental or scientific agency; see discussion above, under heading "Vitamins and Minerals"): 1,200 mg to 2,400 mg (lecithin)

Functions: major source of choline (needed to manufacture the neurotransmitter acetylcholine); speculated benefits include protection against heart disease, memory loss, and nervous-system disease

Food sources: rice, soybeans, cabbage, cauliflower, eggs, garbanzo beans, green beans, lentils, split peas, nuts, organ meats

> 1 egg—2,009 mg
>
> peanut butter, 2 tbsp.—97 mg
>
> cauliflower, 1 cup—107 mg
>
> steak, beef, 3½ oz.—466 mg

Adverse reactions: may include "fishy" body odor, nausea, vomiting, dizziness

Brewer's Yeast

Common dosage (not established or endorsed by any governmental or scientific agency; see discussion above, under heading "Vitamins and Minerals"): brewer's yeast contains B vitamins; therefore, the dosages would be the same as those previously listed under B vitamins.

Functions: supplies B vitamins, protein, and minerals; bulk-forming agent prevents constipation

Sources: tablets, powder, flakes

Adverse reactions: may include nausea, diarrhea

Bioflavenoids

Dosage: none established

Functions: act as antioxidants; often combined with vitamin C

Food sources: pulp and rind of citrus fruits, green peppers, apricots, cherries, papaya, grapes, tomatoes, broccoli

Adverse reactions: none expected; may include diarrhea if taken in high doses

Evening Primrose Oil/Borage Oil/Flaxseed

Common dosage (not established or endorsed by any governmental or scientific agency; see discussion above, under heading "Vitamins and Minerals"): 500 mg to 2,000 mg; 1 tbsp. to 2 tbsp. of ground flaxseed

Functions: contain linolenic and linoleic acids (essential fatty acids needed for the body to function and to make anti-inflammatory compounds); reputed to help menopause symptoms, anxiety, and heart disease

Food sources: ground flax meal, salmon, tuna, sardines, pumpkin seeds, sunflower seeds, walnuts

Adverse reactions: unlikely; however, large amounts of ground flaxseed can cause diarrhea

L-tyrosine
(supplementation is not recommended without medical supervision)

Common dosage (not established or endorsed by any governmental or scientific agency; see discussion above, under heading "Vitamins and Minerals"): 2,000 mg to 3,000 mg

Functions: manufactures neurotransmitters; building block of protein

Food sources: almonds, avocados, bananas, cheese, lima beans, lean meat, turkey, tuna, egg white, soy products

    cottage cheese, low-fat, 1 cup—1,492 mg

    cheddar cheese, 1 oz.—341 mg

    1 egg—257 mg

    yogurt, low-fat, 8 oz.—601 mg

    cod, 3 oz.—655 mg

    mackerel, canned, 1 cup—1,487 mg

    macaroni, protein-fortified, 1 cup—253 mg

    top sirloin, lean, broiled, 3½ oz.—1,020 mg

    skinless chicken, light meat, roasted, 3½ oz.—1,043 mg

Adverse reactions: may include changes in blood pressure, migraine headaches

L-phenylalanine
(Use of supplements is not recommended without medical supervision.)

Common dosage (not established or endorsed by any governmental or scientific agency; see discussion above, under heading "Vitamins and Minerals"): 2,000 mg to 3,000 mg

Functions: manufactures neurotransmitters; building block of protein

Food sources: almonds, avocados, bananas, cheese, lean meats, poultry

cottage cheese, low-fat, 1 cup—1,510 mg

provolone cheese, 1 oz.—697 mg

1 egg—334 mg

snapper, 3 oz.—873 mg

canned tuna, light, in water, 3 oz.—847 mg

chuck roast, lean, braised, 3½ oz.—1,213 mg

skim milk, 1 cup—403 mg

peanut butter, creamy, 2 tbsp.—408 mg

skinless chicken, light meat, roasted, 3½ oz.—1,226 mg

white fish, 3 oz.—812 mg

Adverse reactions: may include changes in blood pressure, migraine headaches

Phosphatidylserine (PS)

Common dosage (not established or endorsed by any governmental or scientific agency; see discussion above, under heading "Vitamins and Minerals"): 100 mg to 200 mg (be sure to use PS derived from soybean lecithin rather than from bovine sources; otherwise, there is a remote possibility of contracting Mad Cow Disease from impure bovine sources)

Functions: essential for healthy cell membranes, especially in the brain; purported to enhance memory and cognitive processes

Food sources: Food contains insignificant amounts of phosphatidylserine; therefore, supplementation usually is required. Foods that contain precursors for the manufacturing of PS include nuts, seeds, grains, green leafy vegetables, fish, flaxseed, eggs, dairy products

Adverse reactions: none expected

Sources for this section: Bowes and Church, Food Values of Portions Commonly Used, *sixteenth edition, Lippincott, 1994;* Dietary Reference Intakes *(chart), Food and Nutrition Board, National Academy of Sciences, 1999, 2000; Sarubin, A.,* The Health Professional's Guide to Popular Dietary Supplements, *American Dietetic Association, 2000.*

Herbs

At some point in time, everyone has used a medicinal herb. Can't remember buying any? When was the last time you took an aspirin for a headache, took Sudafed for hay fever, or drank a few cups of coffee to "perk up"? If you have used any of these products, you have benefited from a healing herb, perhaps without realizing it.

In fact, many of today's medicines are derived from plants or are synthetic reproductions of plants. Aspirin, for example, was originally derived from white willow bark and meadowsweet. The heart medicine digitalis originated from the foxglove plant. Metamucil consists of psyllium. The chemotherapy drugs vincristine and vinblastine came from the Madagascar periwinkle tree; and Taxol, also a chemotherapy drug, is obtained from the bark of the Pacific yew tree.

Prior to World War II, herbal medicines were commonly used by physicians. They were prescribed along with or in place of other medicine. They still are widely incorporated into medical treatment in Europe. The popularity of herbal medicine has waned in this country in favor of the booming pharmaceutical business.

When pharmaceutical companies develop and research drugs that are subject to the time-consuming and costly process of obtaining FDA approval, the companies expect to recoup the expense and turn a profit by holding the patent on the product. Natural substances, however, are not patentable. Because there are no exclusivity rights involved, companies are not as motivated to spend time and money proving an herb's worth by involving it in research studies and by marketing the product.

Times, though, are changing. People are displaying a renewed interest in phytomedicines (plant-based medicines). This does not imply that Americans have rejected Western medical practices. Rather, it means that we now are realizing that herbal preparations can complement medical treatment. When used responsibly, healing herbs are safe and effective alternatives.

Guidelines for Using Herbs

▣ Consult a knowledgeable professional. This usually will be a qualified herbalist, since most physicians and pharmacists are not experts on phytomedicine.

▣ Educate yourself about the herbs you are taking. Just as you would read information about a pharmaceutical drug's actions, dosage, side effects, and contraindications before taking it, you should be equally informed about herbs.

▣ Do not disregard mainstream medicine, especially for the treatment of serious illness. Herbs can be very effective in the prevention of illness, the improvement of symptoms, or the treatment of mild problems. If you intend to use them or are using them to complement your medical regimen, be sure to tell your doctor. Herb–drug interactions do exist.

▣ Do not use herbs indiscriminately. They can be powerful medicines and are worthy of the same respect as pharmaceutical medications.

▣ Unless you are a botanist, gathering your own herbs can be dangerous.

▣ Purchase herbs from reputable companies that have some longevity in the business. This helps to ensure a quality product and reduces the likelihood of adulteration. Contact the manufacturer with any questions you have about the product. Credible companies will welcome inquiries.

▣ Use herbal preparations as directed on the package. Herbs are sold in many forms (capsules, tablets, extracts, powders, tinctures, teas, creams, dried), so dosages and instructions vary. To be safe, start out with the smallest dose and gradually increase the amount you take. Do not exceed the recommended dosage or duration. If taking herbs on an empty stomach induces nausea, try taking them with food. If you experience a severe or allergic reaction, discontinue the herb and seek medical advice.

▣ Check the expiration date, and try to buy your products in a store with good turnover.

▣ As noted in Chapter 2, some herbs are phytohormones. If you are not a candidate for estrogen therapy, you may wish to avoid these preparations as well. However, preliminary research indicates that phytoestrogens do not stimulate breast and uterine tissue in the same way estrogen does. This may be due to the weaker estrogenic activity (1/1,000 of the potency of estrogen).

Commonly Recommended Herbs

Note: Since dosages of herbs depend on the method of administration (tablets, capsules, liquid, etc.), no common dosages are listed here. Follow the directions on the label or consult an herbalist.

Black Cohosh (*Cimicifuga racemosa*)

Uses

▣ Historically, Native Americans used this herb to reduce inflammation (for example, from arthritis or a sore throat), to treat menstrual problems and menopausal symptoms, and to facilitate childbirth.

▣ In Germany, it is the key ingredient in a few of the medicines prescribed for menopausal changes. Remifemin is a derivative of black cohosh that, in a German study, was found to provide symptomatic relief akin to Premarin, a common American brand of HRT.

▣ Some studies, as well as anecdotal information, report that black cohosh relieves most menopausal symptoms.

▣ It has been postulated that black cohosh exerts its effects by binding to the estrogen receptors throughout the body.

Safety/Side Effects

◎ The long-term effects of black cohosh are unknown; therefore, limiting usage to 6 months is prudent.

◎ Long-term data on the safety of Remifemin is lacking, so the German government limits its usage to 6 months.

◎ Side effects are generally rare. Symptoms of toxicity may include dizziness, nausea, diarrhea, headache, visual dimness, and lowered heart rate and blood pressure. It also may enhance the effect of blood-pressure medicine, so consult your physician if you take medicine for high blood pressure.

◎ Black cohosh has been thought to stimulate the body in ways similar to estrogen. However, some recent studies have found that even though black cohosh helps alleviate menopausal symptoms, it doesn't stimulate the body like estrogen. This is still a controversial issue.

Dong Quai (*Angelica sinensis*)

Uses

◎ Dong quai often is referred to as the "female ginseng."

◎ Traditionally, Asian women have used it for a wide range of gynecological problems, such as menstrual irregularities, PMS, and menopause. It also has been used for hypertension and insomnia (it has a mild sedating effect).

◎ Herbalists often use dong quai to quell a variety of menopausal changes, especially hot flashes and night sweats.

◎ Dong quai is not thought to exert an estrogenic effect.

Safety/Side Effects

◎ Dong quai may exert an anticoagulation effect; therefore, if you are taking blood thinners, dong quai is not recommended.

◙ This herb may cause photosensitivity (make you more susceptible to sunburn).

◙ Dong quai generally is not recommended for women with menorrhagia (heavy menses).

Ginseng (*Panax ginseng*)

Uses

◙ Consult a knowledgeable herbalist/naturopath before buying ginseng, because it often is adulterated and mislabeled. There also are different species of panax available (for example, Oriental and American), as well as a different preparation known as eleuthero (for example, Siberian). These products often are confused and used interchangeably when, in fact, their effectiveness varies.

◙ The main active ingredients in ginseng are ginsenosides, and the content of these ingredients should be listed on the label.

◙ Ginseng is believed to be an adaptogen (tonic) that fortifies resistance, supports normal body functions, and improves vitality. It also functions as an antioxidant.

◙ Ginseng may reduce the risk of some types of cancer, including ovarian, esophageal, laryngeal, pancreatic, and stomach.[3]

◙ Ginseng is used by herbalists to relieve menopausal discomforts. It also is reputed to enhance thinking abilities.

◙ Take ginseng early in the day, as it may cause insomnia or jitteriness.

Safety/Side Effects

◙ There are conflicting reports regarding ginseng's estrogenic activity.

◙ The side effects of this herb may include insomnia, nervousness, diarrhea, and increased blood pressure.

▨ Ginseng may exert an anticoagulation effect; therefore, it is not recommended if you are taking a blood thinner. It also can lower blood-sugar levels, so consult your physician if you are diabetic or hypoglycemic.

Chaste Tree (*Vitex agnus-castus*)

Uses

▨ This herb is commonly used in Europe for PMS and menopausal symptoms. It is believed to function as a hormone balancer by increasing levels of progesterone in relation to estrogen.

▨ Anecdotal clinical reports indicate that vitex helps alleviate fluid retention, breast tenderness, hot flashes, vaginal dryness, and mood swings.

Safety/Side Effects

▨ Although rare, side effects may include itching and digestive disturbances.

Damiana (*Turnera diffusa*)

Uses

▨ This herb is reputed to be a sexual stimulant, thereby increasing libido.

▨ Herbalists also use damiana as a general tonic to improve feelings of well-being, and as a laxative.

Safety/Side Effects

▨ Damiana may interfere with iron absorption. Otherwise, when used in low dosages, it is generally regarded as safe. Excessive amounts may be linked to hallucinations and liver injury.

Cranberry (*Vaccinium macrocarpon*)

Uses

▣ In the seventeenth century, cranberry was used to provide relief from stomach ailments, liver problems, scurvy, and cancer. Native Americans used cranberry to make wound dressings.[4]

▣ Today, cranberry is used to prevent urinary tract infections. It is believed to work by preventing bacteria from adhering to the walls of the bladder and urethra.

▣ Many cranberry drinks found in the grocery store are high in sugar and calories, and low in cranberry juice (containing 10 percent to 20 percent real juice). Cranberry juice cocktails contain more real juice (25 percent to 35 percent) and have been found to be effective at the level of 10 ounces per day. Unsweetened cranberry juice is the most potent form and tastes quite tart. It usually is considered too strong and sour to be palatable, but diluting it with water helps.

▣ Cranberry-extract capsules are effective.

Safety/Side Effects

▣ Cranberry juice is beneficial unless you are allergic to it. In large amounts (or if using the unsweetened variety), it may cause gastric irritation or diarrhea.

▣ Avoid large doses if you are on medicine for urinary or kidney problems.

▣ When left untreated, urinary tract infections can cause scarring and damage the kidneys. Be sure to consult a doctor if you suspect an infection.

Uva Ursi (*Arctostaphylos uva ursi*)

Uses

- Also known as bearberry, this herb was traditionally used by the Chinese and Native Americans as a diuretic and urinary antiseptic.

- Today, uva ursi is an ingredient in many herbal diuretics and urinary-tract preparations. It often is used to relieve the pain of bladder infections, as well as for its antibacterial properties.

Safety/Side Effects

- Uva ursi is not as effective as a urinary-tract antiseptic if acidic foods (citrus fruits/juices, sauerkraut) and supplements (vitamin C) are consumed. This is because uva ursi requires alkaline urine to exert its effects.

- Your urine may turn green while using uva ursi.

- If you are on diuretic therapy or being treated for hypertension, congestive heart failure, or kidney disease, do not use this herb without consulting your doctor and an herbalist.

- Stop taking uva ursi if you experience nausea or ringing in the ears.

- When left untreated, urinary tract infections can cause scarring and damage the kidneys. Be sure to consult a doctor if you suspect an infection.

Ginkgo (*Ginkgo biloba*)

Uses

- For thousands of years, Chinese herbalists have used ginkgo for coughs, asthma, and inflammation related to allergies.

- One of ginkgo's mechanisms of action works by affecting platelet aggregation (blood clotting), thereby increasing blood flow to the body.

- There is a large volume of literature demonstrating the efficacy of this herb in increasing blood flow in the brain. This is why it is used to treat memory loss, impaired mental functioning, chronic dizziness (vertigo), and ringing in the ears (tinnitus). It currently is being used in Alzheimer's research, and the preliminary results are encouraging.

- Ginkgo also improves blood flow to the legs, which is why it is used to treat certain circulatory disorders in the legs.

- There is evidence that ginkgo also functions as an antioxidant.

Safety/Side Effects

- If you are taking anticoagulants (blood thinners), be aware that ginkgo inhibits blood clotting. This also should be a consideration if you consume aspirin frequently, since aspirin acts as a blood thinner.

- Be sure the product you are taking is standardized to 24 percent flavone glycosides and 6 percent terpenes (these percentages are recognized as a therapeutic concentration).

- Side effects are rarely reported, but in large doses, ginkgo may cause nausea, vomiting, diarrhea, headache, and dizziness.

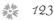

Kava kava (*Piper methysticum*)

Uses

▦ Historically, inhabitants of the South Pacific have made a ritual beverage from kava kava to induce a state of calm and well-being.

▦ Today, this herb is used to treat mild anxiety and stress. It also is useful for insomnia.

▦ A handful of scientific studies have demonstrated kava kava to be a safe and effective alternative to tranquilizing medications such as Valium.

Safety/Side Effects

▦ Recommended usage should not exceed 3 months without medical supervision.

▦ Side effects are uncommon. If they are experienced, they usually are mild and reversible. Side effects may include stomach upset, headache, and dizziness. High doses can produce muscle weakness and visual changes. Extended use may result in a temporary yellowing of the skin. Allergic reactions are rare.

▦ Do not use in conjunction with alcohol, sedatives, narcotics, antianxiety agents, or antidepressants. Do not use if you are suffering from depression.

▦ In responsible doses, use of kava kava may affect motor skills in some people. This should be taken into consideration before driving or operating heavy equipment.

▦ If chronic anxiety or insomnia is experienced, seek professional guidance to determine the underlying cause and to establish a treatment plan.

Valerian (*Valeriana officinalis*)

Uses

❧ Native Americans began using the pulverized roots of the valerian plant to heal wounds.

❧ It traditionally was and currently is used as an antianxiety agent. It "calms the nerves" and can help during times of emotional stress.

❧ Valerian also is used as a sleep aid. Unlike Valium and other tranquilizers, valerian does not cause morning grogginess and is not addictive. However, evaluate how valerian affects you and take this information into consideration before driving or operating heavy equipment.

❧ Valerian has a very distinctive odor, not unlike smelly socks. Do not be alarmed by the unpleasant aroma. It is characteristic of this plant.

Safety/Side Effects

❧ In recommended doses, valerian is regarded as safe.

❧ The effects of using valerian in conjunction with alcohol, sedatives, and narcotics have not been established. Therefore, it is prudent to avoid using valerian with these substances.

❧ If chronic anxiety or insomnia is experienced, seek professional guidance to determine the underlying cause and to establish a treatment plan.

Chamomile
(*Matricaria recutita/Chamaemelum nobile*)

Uses

❧ There are two types of chamomile: German (Hungarian) and Roman (English). Although they are two different plants, their constituents are similar. The German variety is the type most commonly used in the United States.

Perhaps the most well-known feature of chamomile is its ability to induce a state of calm. Many people drink chamomile tea to relax. Since it also appears to stimulate the immune system's ability to fight infection, you may want to drink a cup of tea when feeling under the weather.

Chamomile functions as an antispasmodic, so it is used as a digestive aid to soothe the muscles of the gastrointestinal system.

This herb also has anti-inflammatory and antibacterial properties, and is used topically for wound healing, as well as for treating skin conditions such as eczema.

Safety/Side Effects

Chamomile is considered safe. However, it is prudent to avoid using it with alcohol, sedatives, and narcotics.

Allergic reactions are rare. However, chamomile is a member of the daisy family, so if you are allergic to this classification of plants—which includes ragweed, asters, and chrysanthemums—you may wish to avoid it.

St. John's Wort (*Hypericum perforatum*)

Uses

Wort is an Old English term for "plant," and St. John's wort dates back to the Middle Ages as a remedy for depression and for wound healing (topical use). It also has been used for gastritis and as a diuretic. Today, herbalists use it to treat many of the same ailments.

Recent studies have found St. John's wort to be effective at relieving anxiety and mild to moderate depression (not severe or manic-depressive illness). There is some speculation, supported by preliminary studies, that it may play a role in the treatment of obsessive-compulsive disorder and some eating disorders.

St. John's wort helps to alleviate anxiety and depression by exerting effects of a magnitude similar to antidepressants. Use may continue for as long as 3 months before the full effect of St. John's wort is realized.

Safety/Side Effects

The exact pharmacological mechanism of St. John's wort is unknown. Most theories indicate that it may employ several modes of action, thereby imitating more than one classification of antidepressants. Therefore, it is best not to take St. John's wort with other antidepressants. Since it appears to work, in part, as a selective serotonin reuptake inhibitor—like Prozac, Paxil, or Zoloft—it can be dangerous to combine St. John's wort with a monoamine oxidase (MAO) inhibitor such as Nardil or Parnate. Research on switching from prescription medication to St. John's wort is practically nonexistent. Seek professional advice if you are considering this transition.

St. John's wort may also work, in part, as a MAO inhibitor, so some sources recommend following the same precautions as those outlined for MAO inhibitors. However, more recent sources note that the likelihood of a reaction to St. John's wort is extremely remote and has never been documented. The interaction in question is that MAO inhibitors—in combination with certain foods and medicines—can cause dangerously high blood pressure. These include foods high in tryptophan (such as broad beans) or tyramine (such as aged cheese, wine, beer, avocados, chicken livers, chocolate, bananas, soy sauce, miso soup, tofu, meat tenderizers, salami, bologna), large amounts of caffeine, and medications such as amphetamines, diet pills, narcotics, and cold/hay-fever preparations.

◉ Be sure the product you select is standardized to 0.3 percent hypericin and 3 percent hyperforin (these percentages are recognized as a therapeutic concentration).

◉ St. John's wort may cause photosensitivity (susceptibility to sunburn). To protect against this, avoid prolonged exposure to sunlight, and use sunscreen, especially when taking other photosensitizing drugs.

◉ If you suffer from persistent anxiety or depression, seek professional help. Not only is it crucial to establish a diagnosis, but medication works best when accompanied by counseling.

Guidelines for Common Sudden-Menopausal Changes

The following sample guidelines are set up using a stepwise approach. Try the suggestions listed under step 1 for 2 weeks. If you need further relief from symptoms, continue following the recommendations under step 1 and move on to step 2. After 4 more weeks of steps 1 and 2, incorporate step 3 into the mix. The final step includes herbs (step 2 under anxiety and depression) and should be used for 1 month before seeking additional strategies.

If you require higher vitamin doses or different herbs from those listed below, consult a naturopathic practitioner or herbalist. Keep in mind that some products contain these herbs in combination. If you use a combination product, try to locate one that contains low dosages of each herb.

Hot Flashes/Night Sweats

Step 1:

Vitamin E, 400 IU per dose, 1–2 doses per day

Calcium, 500–600 mg per dose, 2–3 doses per day

Magnesium, 400 mg daily

Vitamin C, 500 mg per dose, 1–2 doses per day

Step 2:

Ground flaxseed, 1–2 tbsp. daily OR soy food, 1–2 servings daily (30–60 mg isoflavones)

Step 3:

Black cohosh, 80 mg per dose, 2 doses per day OR chaste tree (Vitex), 20–40 mg daily OR dong quai, 500 mg daily

Note: For hot flashes and night sweats, take half of the daily dosage (or food servings) in the morning, and half in the evening.

Vaginal Dryness

Step 1:

Vitamin E, 400 IU per dose, 1–2 doses per day; also, vitamin E cream (vaginally) daily, according to package directions

Step 2:

Ground flaxseed, 1–2 tbsp. daily OR soy food, 1–2 servings daily (30–60 mg isoflavones)

Step 3:

Black cohosh, 80 mg per dose, 2 doses per day OR chaste tree (Vitex), 20–40 mg daily

Anxiety/Mood Swings

Step 1:

B-100-B-complex, 1 daily

Vitamin C, 500 mg per dose, 1–2 doses per day

Calcium, 500–600 mg per dose, 2–3 doses per day

Magnesium, 400 mg daily

Step 2:

Kava kava, 150–300 mg per dose, 2 doses per day (equivalent of 50–240 mg of kava pyrones) <u>OR</u> Bach Rescue Remedy, 4 drops per dose, 1–4 doses per day

Depression

Step 1:

B-100-B-complex, 1 daily

Vitamin C, 500 mg per dose, 1–2 doses per day

Ground flaxseed, 1–2 tbsp. daily

Step 2:

St. John's wort, 300 mg per dose, 1–3 doses per day (standardized to 0.3 percent hypericin and 3 percent hyperforin)

Cognitive Changes

Step 1:

B-100-B-complex, 1 daily

Vitamin E, 400 IU per dose, 1–2 doses per day

Vitamin C, 500 mg per dose, 1–2 doses per day

Lecithin, 1,200 mg per dose, 1–2 doses per day

Coenzyme Q10, 50–100 mg daily

Phosphatidylserine, 100 mg per dose, 2 doses per day

Step 2:

Ground flaxseed, 1–2 tbsp. daily <u>OR</u> soy food, 1–2 servings
   daily (30–60 mg isoflavones)

Step 3:

Ginkgo biloba, 40 mg per dose, 2–3 doses per day
   (standardized to 24 percent flavone glycosides and 6 percent
   terpenes)

Chapter Highlights

⚙ Before using dietary supplements, scrutinize your diet. It
should be rich in whole grains and include at least five
servings of fruits and vegetables each day, as well as at least
50 grams of protein. If you need help in evaluating your
eating habits and determining the proper amounts of
proteins, carbohydrates, and fats in your diet, consult a
registered dietitian.

⚙ After deciding which supplements you want to try, gradually
add them one at a time at one-week intervals. If you have
difficulty deciding what to buy, consult a qualified herbalist
or naturopath.

⚙ Buy high-quality standardized herbs from a company that has
longevity in the business. Consult a qualified herbalist or
naturopath if you need guidance when using herbs.

⚙ Keep in mind that no "one size fits all" approach exists to
using dietary supplements. You may have to experiment a
little until you find a regimen that works for you.

⚙ Stay abreast of new information on dietary supplements as it
becomes available.

⚙ Although side effects are relatively uncommon when using
supplements responsibly, be sure to stop taking them and

consult a knowledgeable professional if you experience any side effects.

Doc Talk

▨ Let your physician know which dietary supplements you are taking, as well as the doses of each supplement.

▨ If you are on medication, talk to your doctor and pharmacist about potential supplement-medication interactions.

▨ It is crucial that, for at least two weeks prior to any invasive procedure or surgery, you stop taking any supplements that prolong bleeding time. Discuss this with your doctor before scheduling the test or operation.

▨ Meet with the anesthesiologist prior to any procedure or surgery that requires anesthesia, and inform him/her of any vitamins or herbs you may be taking. Some herbs interact with anesthesia, and it can be dangerous to combine the two.

6

The Hormone Hype

"How do I know if I should go on hormones?" asked 38-year-old *LYNN*. Even though she was a librarian, the volume of information she unearthed on hormone replacement therapy left her feeling confused. Her search for answers began shortly after she opted for a hysterectomy with BSO, a last-ditch effort to treat her endometriosis. Although her menstrual pain subsided after surgery, she began suffering from hot flashes and night sweats. Because the tissue that grows on the pelvic organs during endometriosis is fueled by estrogen, her doctor wanted her to abstain from hormone replacement therapy for several months. She used that time to educate herself about using postmenopausal hormones. She said, "I'm no further ahead now than I was when I began searching for answers."

It's true that information is knowledge; still, people need assistance in making sense of it all. Together, Lynn and I sorted through the data and listed key points that she needed to consider before making an informed decision.

Of the many decisions women make on a daily basis, whether or not to go on hormone replacement therapy (HRT) is one of the most grueling. I frequently hear women voice their ambivalence about whether to try HRT. This issue has overwhelmed many women because they are bombarded with conflicting information almost daily.

Some women are afraid they will end up old and crippled if they don't go on HRT. Others are afraid they will die of breast cancer if they do go on HRT. Almost all fail to realize that the reality lies somewhere in between, and that the decision is theirs alone and is different for everyone.

Women are capable of making this decision for themselves. The secret to digesting the information on hormone replacement therapy is to break it down into bite-size pieces and analyze it within the context of your own symptoms, personal risk factors, and family history.

Addressing symptoms includes identifying your menopausal changes and gauging their severity. Are they tolerable, or do they interfere with your personal or professional life? Do alternatives to hormones exist to help alleviate your symptoms? (See Chapter 2.) Are you willing to invest time into exploring these options and modifying your lifestyle?

An assessment of your personal and family medical history includes determining any medical conditions with which you have been diagnosed, as well as evaluating your risk for osteoporosis, heart disease, cancer, and Alzheimer's disease. Can you break your unhealthy habits and add healthy new ones to lower your risk of developing osteoporosis and heart disease? (See Chapters 3 and 4.) Would the results of specific tests—such as a bone-density scan or a lipid profile—help to make the decision easier? Have you had an estrogen-dependent cancer, or do you have a strong family history of this type of cancer? Have you experienced a sudden menopause at an early age?

These are some of the questions you and your health-care provider should discuss when considering HRT. The answers also need to be balanced against your quality of life. If you have decided against taking hormones or are told you are not a good candidate for them but feel you have exhausted other options, and if you are still so miserable that you are thinking, "What kind of a life is this?"—then you may want to reevaluate your decision. For example, consider using "natural" (bio-identical) hormones in the lowest doses and the safest delivery system for an appropriate length of time and under close supervision to alleviate specific symptoms. Depending on the condition that led to your sudden menopause, this may not be a decision that all physicians endorse, but as long as you enter into it having considered the benefit–risk ratio, it is an informed decision.

Suddenly menopausal women especially need to be proactive and talk to their doctors about a prudent approach to hormone replacement therapy. Remember, every woman's situation is different, and you owe it to yourself to explore all of the options. Be aware that with a sudden menopause, too often a woman isn't really given a choice. If her doctor feels she is a candidate for hormones, she is usually "told" that she will be placed on HRT after the hysterectomy. If the doctor thinks HRT would be risky or unnecessary, he may "tell" her that she isn't a candidate. Women need to know that they should be included in the decision-making process. Woman also need to know that quality of life is just as important as length of life.

Estrogen

Although the word estrogen implies a single substance, three active forms of estrogen have been identified: estrone (E_1), estradiol (E_2), and estriol (E_3). A potent estrogen produced by the ovaries, 17-beta estradiol, is the dominant type of estrogen in premenopausal women. Women who go on HRT and request "natural hormones" usually are referring to estradiol, because it is identical to the type produced in the body. Brand names include Estrace and the transdermal (patch) forms such as Estraderm, Climara, and Vivelle. You also may purchase the generic form under the name estradiol.

For the purposes of this book, when I refer to "natural hormones," I mean the type that is identical to what the ovaries produce (bio-identical), or 17-beta estradiol, implied by the term estradiol. This is different from some of the altered or synthetic versions of estradiol, such as ethinyl estradiol.

Estrone also is a potent estrogen that is produced in the body from the conversion of estradiol. During perimenopause in naturally menopausal women, the secretion of estradiol begins to decline; after menopause, it stops almost entirely. Estrone then becomes the predominant form of estrogen in postmenopausal women. Brand names of estrone include Premarin, Ogen, and Ortho-Est. Premarin is by far the most frequently prescribed hormone. In addition to minute amounts of human estrogens, it contains equine (horse) estrogens.

Estriol is a weak estrogen produced in smaller quantities by the ovaries. It also can be derived from plant sources. Because of its botanical origins, it is not patentable. Although it is not commercially available, it can be obtained by prescription from pharmacies that specialize in compounding medications.

Estriol seems to be very effective in the treatment of vaginal and urinary symptoms, especially vaginal dryness. Since estriol helps to maintain the delicate balance within the urogenital system, it may be especially helpful in women prone to vaginal and urinary tract infections.

Use of estriol does not appear to cause endometrial hyperplasia, a precursor to uterine cancer. Some proponents of estriol speculate that it does not stimulate breast tissue, as do estradiol and estrone. Nor does estriol seem to confer protective benefits to the bones and heart, but only time and continued research will tell.

Keep in mind that although the ovaries warehouse most of a woman's sex hormones, supplemental amounts are produced via chemical reaction by the adrenal glands and fat tissue. So if your ovaries have been removed or have been rendered inactive, you will not be totally devoid of sex hormones, but you will have significantly lower levels.

Advantages of Estrogen

Symptomatic Relief
As described in Chapter 2, taking estrogen can relieve many of the symptoms women experience during a sudden menopause. The

symptoms may not disappear completely, but an improvement usually is noted.

Problems that respond well to estrogen include hot flashes, night sweats, vaginal dryness, atrophic vaginitis, chronic urinary irritations and infections, emotional difficulties, and cognitive changes. Other benefits that may accompany hormone usage are increased feelings of well-being, stability of sleep patterns, and increased oil production in the skin.

Osteoporosis

By far, one of estrogen's strongest attributes is that it enhances calcium absorption and drastically reduces bone loss. Some sources report that estrogen cuts the risk of osteoporosis by 50 percent.

As women are living longer, osteoporosis is becoming a greater threat to our long-term health. This is especially true for women who undergo sudden menopause and lose most of their estrogen at an earlier age than most naturally menopausal women. Chapter 3 explains that osteoporosis results from a cumulative calcium deficiency that develops over a lifetime. However, it is never too late to put a halt to bone loss, especially since osteoporosis is a painful, debilitating disease that bears a tremendous impact on the quality of a woman's remaining years. It can mean the difference between remaining active or becoming bedridden.

Heart Disease

Heart disease, like osteoporosis, should be an issue of concern for women of all ages, especially since poor dietary and exercise habits often are established early in life. However, estrogen plays a pivotal role in heart health, too. Estrogen has been proven—most recently by the Postmenopausal Estrogen/Progestin Interventions trial (PEPI)—to slash a woman's risk of heart disease. In fact, meta-analyses of observational studies suggest a 50 percent reduction. When women experience sudden menopause, especially at an early age, the cardioprotective effects of estrogen are swiftly withdrawn.

Levels of HDL—the "good" cholesterol—increased in all PEPI treatment groups, regardless of the hormone regimen to which they were assigned. Women with hysterectomies had HDL levels that were, on average, greater at the end of the study than the levels of participants in other groups. This was attributed to their ability to take unopposed (without progestin) estrogen because endometrial cancer was not a concern. LDL—"bad" cholesterol— and fibrinogen (the blood-clotting factor associated with strokes and heart attacks) levels decreased in all treatment groups, but triglyceride levels increased.

Recall from Chapter 4 the Heart and Estrogen/Progestin Replacement Study (HERS) results. Initially, the study clouded the estrogen-cardioprotection issue, because it showed a 50 percent increase in the risk of heart attack during the first year of HRT use. After the first year, the risk gradually declined. Keep in mind, though, that the women in this study had advanced heart disease and were placed on both estrogen and progestin because they had not undergone hysterectomies. Again, it is vital that a sudden menopausal woman's cardiac status be evaluated to rule out advanced heart disease before she is placed on HRT.

Alzheimer's Disease

Research into the estrogen-Alzheimer's link is yielding fascinating results. There is compelling evidence suggesting that estrogen may lower the risk of Alzheimer's disease. Furthermore, estrogen replacement therapy appears to delay the onset and slow the progression of the disease in those stricken with Alzheimer's. Not only does this further establish the relationship between estrogen and mental functioning, but if future studies consistently yield the same results, perhaps it will unseat Alzheimer's as the number-one cause of dementia in elderly women.

Colon Cancer

Although some data regarding colon cancer and the use of HRT are conflicting, recent studies are encouraging. It seems that exogenous estrogen (estrogen taken as a supplement, rather than produced within the body) may confer protection and reduce the risk of colon cancer. Hopefully, further research into this relationship will yield similar results.

Disadvantages of Estrogen

Endometrial Cancer

It has long been known that unopposed estrogen therapy (taking estrogen without progesterone/progestin) increases the likelihood of developing uterine cancer. That is why this therapy commonly is given only to women who have undergone hysterectomies. A woman with an intact uterus generally is prescribed estrogen with progesterone/progestin, which lowers the risk of endometrial cancer. If the combination therapy is not used, annual transvaginal ultrasound tests or endometrial biopsies are necessary to monitor for hyperplasia (endometrial overgrowth).

Breast Cancer

The ravages of battling anorexia nervosa for many years left 29-year-old SYLVIA in the midst of sudden menopause. Besides wanting to treat her night sweats and vaginal dryness, her physician was extremely concerned about her bone density. In addition to the anorexia's depriving her body of essential nutrients, being estrogen deficient at such an early age was detrimental to her bone health. Although Sylvia wanted to feel better and certainly didn't want to develop osteoporosis, her primary concern was breast cancer. She told me, "I don't want to take anything that will cause cancer."

After discussing the pros and cons with me and her doctor, she decided to use HRT on a short-term basis (less than 10 years). This would afford her bones protection during the years when her body was still capable of building bone. It would also alleviate her night sweats and vaginal dryness. Each year she plans to reevaluate her decision with her doctor. She may decide on another approach in light of any new information available.

───◄═•═►───

The risk of breast cancer has to be the number-one reason why women hesitate to go on HRT. Of the dozens of studies that have been conducted, there still is no conclusive answer about the impact of estrogen on breast cancer. Some studies indicate that HRT increases the risk (and of these studies, some correlate the risk to the number of years using HRT), and others indicate that HRT decreases the risk.

For example, the Nurses' Health Study showed that the risk of breast cancer increased 50 percent in women using post-menopausal hormones for 5 years or longer.[1] However, another, similar study failed at all to demonstrate this increase in risk. In fact, it concluded that a reduced risk of breast cancer existed in HRT users of longer than 8 years.[2]

It is known that estrogen stimulates the proliferation of breast cells and fuels estrogen-dependent tumors. For this reason, HRT usually is not recommended for women at high risk for breast cancer or for those with a history of estrogen-dependent breast tumors.

However, some physicians recently have been prescribing HRT for a select group of breast cancer survivors. Typically, these are women diagnosed with early-stage, nonestrogen-dependent, lymph node-negative breast tumors who have been cancer free for at least 2 years. A few doctors are even using hormones in women with early-stage, estrogen-dependent, lymph node–negative breast tumors who have been cancer free for at least 5 years. Obviously, close surveillance of these women is necessary to determine the benefits and risks of this approach.

In light of the conflicting evidence, I believe women need to be aware of the possibility of a direct link, even though a definitive answer does not yet exist. In other words, the jury is still out on the link between HRT and increased risk of breast cancer.

Methods of Administration

There are several different ways to obtain exogenous estrogen. I believe this selection is a bonus, because it provides women with options. No single prescription of estrogen works for everyone. Some women do better with the transdermal (patch) delivery system, while others prefer tablets.

If you fail to experience adequate relief on your hormone regimen, do not give up. You may simply require a different delivery route, type of estrogen, or dosage. If what is commercially available at your local pharmacy does not suit your needs, there are compounding pharmacies that can tailor the hormones to your body's specifications. You, your doctor, and the pharmacist will need to work together closely to monitor the effectiveness of the hormone regimen and to make adjustments as needed.

SHANNON, a 39-year-old realtor, underwent a hysterectomy with BSO due to years of unexplained heavy menstrual bleeding. It was so severe that it left her anemic and housebound for 2 weeks of every month. She was placed on Premarin postoperatively to prevent hot flashes and to confer protection to her bones and heart. Two months after surgery, she announced her plans to discontinue using Premarin.

When I questioned her about this decision, she cited the side effects of headaches and nausea as her reason for not wanting to use estrogen. She said that she would rather take her chances with the hot flashes. After I explained to her that not all estrogen preparations elicit the same side effects and I presented her with all of the options, she decided to give the patch a try. Her doctor prescribed the lowest dosage of Climara available to reduce the likelihood of side effects. The patch also had the advantage of utilizing a different route of administration and a different type of estrogen from the Premarin. This approach was perfect for Shannon. She was able to achieve good control of her menopausal symptoms without experiencing headaches or nausea.

More often than not, finding the perfect "recipe" for any individual is a gradual process, so be patient. Also, keep in mind that women in their 20s and 30s who undergo sudden menopause and who are candidates for estrogen may require higher dosages than women in their 40s and 50s, who are closer to the time of natural menopause. This is because women in their 20s and 30s have higher hormone levels naturally. As we age, our hormone levels gradually decline. Otherwise, it is generally recommended to stick with the lowest dosage needed to relieve symptoms while providing protection against osteoporosis and heart disease.

Oral

Not all oral estrogens are created equal. However, they do share the characteristic of having a more appreciable effect on increasing HDL levels than do other forms of estrogen.

I sometimes hear a woman say, "I tried Premarin but still had side effects. I guess I just can't take the pill form." This is not necessarily true. The problem usually has more to do with the predominant type of estrogen contained in the tablet and the individual's response to it. Some forms may relieve your symptoms, while other forms may not. Some forms may cause headaches, breast tenderness, or depression, while others may not.

Premarin certainly is not the only oral estrogen available, but it is the most commonly prescribed, is the type most frequently used in research, and has been commercially available for decades. It also is heavily marketed to physicians and consumers. Premarin belongs to a classification of hormones called conjugated—or mixed—estrogens. Specifically, this drug contains conjugated equine estrogens, which are derived from pregnant mares' urine (hence the name Premarin).

Some women feel perfectly fine while taking Premarin, and other women do not. Some experts attribute this inconsistency to the fact that our bodies respond to and metabolize horse-derived hormones differently from how they respond to hormones produced by our own ovaries.

This may be easier to understand if you think of our hormone receptors as locks and our hormones as keys. Our bodily organs are coated with estrogen receptors that need to bond with the estrogen our bodies produce in order to prevent the menopausal symptoms that women report. From puberty to menopause, the most biologically active estrogen is 17-beta estradiol. At adequate levels, it circulates through the bloodstream and bonds with the receptors, just as a key would fit into a lock. A type of estrogen that is foreign to our bodies—for example, equine estrogen, which is specific to horses—might be a key that jams the lock, increasing the possibility of side effects.

Alternatively, the estrogen 17-beta estradiol is available orally in both the generic form and as the brand Estrace. These medications may be purchased at your local pharmacy. As I noted previously, this is the exact type of estrogen to which our bodies are accustomed.

In my experience, women feel better on this type of estrogen; however, everyone is different. If you are taking conjugated estrogens and are experiencing side effects, you may respond better to 17-beta estradiol. Compounding pharmacies can formulate estradiol in the dosage and form that you need, as well as combine it with other hormones.

Some estrogen tablets primarily contain estrone, the form of estrogen that predominates after menopause. Estrone is produced in the ovaries and by adipose (fat) tissue. Premarin contains estrone, as it is a mixed estrogen. Ogen and Ortho-Est mainly supply estrone. If residual symptoms persist when taking these preparations, it may be due to the lower levels of estradiol.

Since estriol is the weakest form of estrogen, it has been largely overlooked until recently. Special compounding pharmacies, such as Madison Pharmacy Associates, supply estriol in a variety of forms. Estriol is tailored to an individual's needs and may be prepared alone or in combination with progesterone, testosterone, estradiol, and estrone. For example, Madison Pharmacy Associates makes Bi-Estrogen, which contains 80 percent estriol and 20 percent estradiol. Tri-Estrogen is a combination of the three human estrogens, with the largest percentage being estriol (80 percent estriol, 10 percent estradiol, 10 percent estrone). Although these are yet other options for women, especially those with mild symptoms or for when HRT is to be used with caution, they have not gained great acceptance within the medical community, perhaps because research is scanty.

Transdermal

For women who cannot tolerate oral estrogen because it aggravates certain preexisting medical conditions—such as gallbladder disease, hypertension, or migraine headaches—the transdermal method (the patch) may be an effective solution. It avoids the "hepatic first-pass effect" because the estrogen is delivered directly into the bloodstream without first passing through the liver. This is not as taxing to the digestive organs and liver, thereby eliminating the reason some women cannot tolerate it. Because it bypasses the liver, the patch does not have as potent an effect on raising HDL levels as oral estrogens do. However, preliminary data on its cardioprotective effects, as well as on its bone-preserving capabilities, are encouraging and parallel the effects from orally administered estrogen.

The transdermal delivery system provides estradiol at a controlled rate through the skin. Brand names include Estraderm, Climara, Vivelle, and Fem Patch. These products resemble a round Band-Aid and release estrogen while adhering to the skin. Most women wear the patch on the abdomen (avoid the area where the waistband falls, because it may rub and become irritated), but if you have sensitive skin, the back or hips may work better for you. Since the sites should be rotated, you probably will try them all. Depending on the brand, the patch needs to be changed once to twice a week. For this reason, it is convenient for people who have a hard time remembering to take medicine daily.

A suddenly menopausal woman who has a uterus needs to use progesterone with the estrogen. Only one patch exists that combines the two, and it doesn't include the natural form of progesterone. Any woman may use the patch, but women with a uterus need to use progesterone/progestin. This can be in the form of a tablet or cream or any of the other methods of administration. Since hysterectomized women don't need progesterone, the patch is a desirable delivery method and is very convenient for them (i.e., they don't have to remember to take any other pill).

Many women are pleased with the patch and find that it provides effective relief of menopausal changes. Some are dissatisfied because the patch falls off easily, especially in a humid environment. Although it can be reattached, some women find this bothersome. If this occurs, you may want to try a different brand of the patch. In addition, a skin allergy to the adhesive may develop.

An alternative to the patch is estrogen absorbed via the skin in cream or gel form. Compounding pharmacies can supply the various types of estrogen—alone or in combination with progesterone—as a cream or gel. As a general rule, these products need to be applied once or twice daily.

Vaginal Creams

Estrogen comes in a cream form that is inserted into the vagina using a measured applicator. Although some of the medication is absorbed into the bloodstream, it mostly influences the cells that line the vagina and urethra. This helps to strengthen those tissues and to correct vaginal dryness and irritation, as well as to decrease inflammation of the urethra. These predominantly localized effects are why vaginal estrogen creams are recommended for urogenital changes only.

In commonly prescribed dosages, vaginal cream probably will not alleviate other menopausal symptoms such as hot flashes, mood swings, or mental changes, and you should not rely on it to foster a healthy heart or bones. However, nor does it aggravate preexisting medical conditions such as gallbladder disease, hypertension, or thrombophlebitis. Brand names for vaginal estrogen cream include Estrace, Premarin, and Ogen.

Compounding pharmacies also make estriol vaginal suppositories. Recall from earlier in this chapter that estriol is particularly effective for vaginal and urinary-tract problems. These preparations are used daily to several times a week and may be tapered off, depending on the dosage and the severity of the urogenital changes.

Other Forms

Estrogen can be administered in a few other ways as well. Estradiol vaginal rings are now available for use in the United States.

Once the ring is anchored into the vagina, it remains there for 90 days. While in place, the ring continuously releases a small amount of estradiol. This is effective for localized symptoms of urogenital atrophy—vaginal dryness and itching—as well as urinary urgency and discomfort. The brand name is Estring.

Monthly injections are no longer commonly used, mainly because of the availability of other forms of estrogen. However, this method is a reliable source of estrogen. Sometimes, injections are used postoperatively in women whose ovaries have been removed. This is especially the case for younger women, who would be the ones most likely to feel the effects of a plummeting estrogen level more immediately and severely. The injection is a good way of obtaining a therapeutic level of estrogen quickly.

Other delivery systems exist that are either new or have not yet received FDA approval. These include subcutaneous estrogen pellets, which are implanted beneath the skin; buccal estrogen, which is placed in the mouth and dissolves into the cheek; and estrogen gel that is rubbed into the skin.

Progesterone

In a woman who has had a hysterectomy, a progestational agent (something that readies the system for pregnancy, such as the hormone progesterone) generally is not prescribed. This is because progesterone's principal benefit is to protect the uterus from overstimulation by estrogen, with the subsequent risk of endometrial cancer. On the other hand, some hysterectomized women do use progesterone, so that their HRT more closely simulates their body's preoperative hormonal environment. If you have undergone a sudden menopause but have retained your uterus, adding progesterone/progestin is a must, because it protects the uterus from cancer.

Progesterone is a term that is used loosely. It has come to encompass both the natural and the synthetic forms of the hormone. Although referring to all progestational agents as progesterone probably has evolved out of convenience, natural progesterone should be distinguished from its synthetic counterpart.

Progesterone is one of the naturally occurring hormones produced by the ovaries during the luteal phase of the menstrual cycle. It is referred to as the hormone of pregnancy, as it literally means "for gestation."

As an exogenous hormone, progesterone is derived from Mexican or South American wild yams and soybeans. This substance is identical to the chemical messenger produced by the ovaries monthly. That is why it is referred to as "natural" (bio-identical) even though it is synthesized in a laboratory.

Progestins, on the other hand, are synthetic hormones that are derivatives of natural progesterone. Pharmaceutical companies alter the chemical structure of progesterone so that, as progestin, it takes on other properties. Progestins are used in oral contraceptives, as well as in HRT. Examples are medroxyprogesterone acetate, Provera, Cycrin, norgestimate, and norethindrone acetate.

While some women tolerate progestin well, others are sensitive to its slight chemical difference from progesterone. This can result in side effects or PMS-type symptoms. Sometimes lowering the dosage of progestin alleviates these side effects; however, this does not always work. In such cases, women may benefit from micronized progesterone. In fact, more women using HRT are starting off with progesterone rather than trying it as a last resort.

Women with allergies to peanuts should be aware that most micronized, natural progesterone is formulated in a peanut-oil base. Do not use these products if you are allergic to peanuts.

Advantages of Progesterone

Symptomatic Relief

Progesterone/progestin can alleviate hot flashes. This regimen typically is used in women with vasomotor symptoms for whom estrogen is not recommended. Mayo Clinic researchers found that using megestrol acetate, a synthetic progestin, reduced the frequency and severity of hot flashes in women—as well as in men being treated for prostate cancer—85 percent of the time.[3] Other studies have borne out similar results.

Uterine Cancer

In the 1960s and 1970s, unopposed estrogen (without a progestational agent) often was prescribed in high doses in women who still had their uterus. This led to higher rates of uterine cancer, because taking estrogen in this manner can cause excessive buildup of the uterine lining, a condition called hyperplasia. Sometimes, this condition progresses to cancer.

Uterine cancer always goes through a hyperplastic phase, but hyperplasia does not always progress to cancer. For this reason, a progestational agent is added to estrogen therapy. It precipitates the clean and regular sloughing off of the estrogen-induced proliferation of the uterine lining, resulting in a "period" and preventing buildup of the endometrium.

Once you have discovered the perfect balance of estrogen and progesterone/progestin for you, your menstrual flow should be somewhat lighter than that of your natural menses. Eventually, it will disappear. Persistent, excessively heavy or irregular bleeding should be brought to your doctor's attention. If tests—such as transvaginal ultrasound, aspiration biopsy, or D&C—show that you have hyperplasia, you probably will be prescribed a few months of progestin alone, which usually resolves the problem.

Osteoporosis

Until recently, the contribution of progesterone/progestin to preventing osteoporosis was overlooked. Attention was focused on estrogen because it nullified the breakdown of bone. However, progesterone/progestin now has assumed its rightful place in maintaining the bone balance. Studies have shown progesterone/progestin to stimulate bone-building activity. For this reason, some hysterectomized women opt to add a progestational agent to their estrogen therapy.

Disadvantages of Progesterone

Withdrawal Bleeding

Imagine *KIM's* shock when her menstrual cycles suddenly stopped at the age of 33. Diagnosed with premature ovarian failure (a condition of undetermined origin that results in the cessation of menstrual cycles before the age of 40), she entered into a sudden menopause. Given her age, she opted for HRT. She automatically assumed that since her period had stopped of its own accord, she would not have to deal with it again. However, her doctor placed her on a regimen of medication that induced withdrawal bleeding. Since she considered being amenorrheic (without menstrual periods) the only perk of the premature ovarian failure, she was unhappy about the withdrawal bleeding. Once she brought this to her doctor's attention, he switched her to a daily combined regimen of hormones. Seven months later, she no longer experienced any bleeding.

One aspect of menopause that most women eagerly embrace is the cessation of their monthly cycles. Imagine their dismay when they realize that taking HRT—especially in the cyclical fashion (taking estrogen for a given number of days, followed by a combination of estrogen and a progestational agent)—means the resumption of monthly bleeding. Of course, hysterectomized women do not experience this, no matter which hormone regimen they take.

This reactivation of endometrial activity discourages many women from trying or remaining on hormones. To help alleviate this annoyance, alternatives to the cyclical dosing schedule have been created. For example, continuous combined therapy involves taking smaller daily doses of both estrogen and a progestational agent. Theoretically, women would become amenorrheic (without menses) under such a regimen. Although eventually most women stop bleeding, this normally does not happen right away. In the meantime, the occurrence of any bleeding may be erratic and unscheduled.

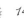

Wyeth-Ayerst, the manufacturer of Prempro—Premarin and Cycrin combined into a tablet and taken daily—reported that in studies using Prempro, 22.7 percent of women were amenorrheic for the entire year of the study, and 53.3 percent experienced amenorrhea during the last 4 months of the study. They did bleed for the first 8 months. This continuous combination therapy also can be accomplished by using CombiPatch. This transdermal system combines estradiol with a synthetic progestin.

Another dosing schedule that exists for women who want to avoid monthly bleeding is using estrogen monthly and adding the progestational agent on a quarterly basis. However, this also may result in irregular and heavy bleeding. Keep in mind that the longer a woman has been postmenopausal, the less likely it is that she will experience bleeding.

Heart Disease

It once was thought that adding progesterone/progestin to estrogen replacement therapy completely nullified the cardioprotective effect of the estrogen. However, the PEPI Trial has disputed this belief. This study found that although unopposed estrogen was the optimal regimen for raising HDL levels, combining it with a progestational agent still improved the levels. Interestingly, combining estrogen with micronized progesterone ran a close second in cardioprotection to taking estrogen alone. Given this information, along with the risk of endometrial cancer, a woman with an intact uterus needs to take a progestational agent, and natural progesterone would be a wise choice.

Breast Cancer

As with estrogen, the effects of progesterone/progestin on breast cells are unclear. Although no conclusive evidence exists to indicate that estrogen is a direct cause of breast cancer, estrogen does cause breast cells to proliferate. A progestational agent is thought to protect against this breast-stimulating activity, although this, too, is debatable. Since there is no clear-cut answer to hormone usage and breast cancer, I have listed it under disadvantages.

Methods of Administration

Just as there are different ways to administer estrogen, there are various vehicles for delivering progestational agents. As with estrogen, there is no blanket prescription that covers everyone. Treatment is aimed at finding an adequate dosage to protect the uterus with the fewest possible side effects.

Various schedules for taking progesterone/progestin also exist (see Table 6.5). For example, it may be administered cyclically with estrogen. A typical regimen would be to take estrogen for 21 to 25 days per month and then to add a progestational agent for 7 to 12 days of that same time frame. Withdrawal bleeding would occur during the week that no hormones were used.

As mentioned previously, continuous therapy also is an option. This may mean using both estrogen and progesterone/progestin daily, or using estrogen on a daily basis with an intermittent progestational agent 12 to 14 days per month. You and your health care provider can decide on a schedule that is best suited for your needs. If after 3 months you are dissatisfied, some fine-tuning or another regimen may be in order.

Oral

Most women who need a progestational agent are prescribed a synthetic version (medroxyprogesterone acetate) in the form of Provera or Cycrin. Other oral progestins include Curretab, Amen, and Aygestin.

Ingesting separate tablets of estrogen and progestin allows for easier manipulation of dosages, especially if you've just begun HRT and are in trial-and-error mode with your doctor. However, Premarin and Cycrin have been formulated into a one-tablet system, which may be more convenient.

Premphase consists of .625 mg of Premarin for a 28-day cycle, plus 5 mg of Cycrin for 14 days. Prempro consists of .625 mg of Premarin plus 2.5 mg or 5 mg of Cycrin daily. Currently, these are the only dosages available in the combination blister packs.

Recently there has been an explosion of one-tablet systems entering the market. These tablets combine estrogen with progestin. Some of these preparations use estradiol with a synthetic progestin—Ortho-Prefest, for example—and others use a synthetic version of estradiol with a synthetic progestin—for example, femhrt. The latter resembles low-dose birth-control pills.

Although side effects can be experienced with estrogens, they are more likely to occur with progestins. Common side effects include bloating, breast tenderness, headache, and mood changes.

Some women find that they simply cannot tolerate the synthetic version, even in the lowest dose. This may be true if they were prone to PMS premenopausally. It is not unusual for women to say, "I just don't like the way I feel on it." Sometimes, switching to natural progesterone helps.

Natural micronized progesterone obtained from a compounding pharmacy does come in tablet form. When taken orally, the liver rapidly metabolizes much of the progesterone before it reaches the tissues; therefore, higher, more frequent doses may be needed throughout the day. Recently, natural micronized progesterone has become commercially available. It is manufactured under the brand name Prometrium and can be obtained at your local pharmacy.

Depending on the type of oral preparation compounded at the pharmacy, taking it two to three times a day may be necessary. The even-release tablets help to prevent the "peak and trough" response—thereby requiring fewer daily doses—as well as the drowsy feeling that may stem from natural progesterone.

Topical

Progesterone cream is readily absorbed through the skin and delivered into the bloodstream. Like estrogen patches, topical progesterone avoids passing through the liver first, the so-called hepatic first-pass effect. If this delivery system is chosen, you simply rub the prescribed amount into a fatty area of your body (abdomen, hips, etc.) for the required number of days.

When a compounding pharmacy formulates the cream for you, the pharmacist and your doctor will determine the specific amount and the duration of usage. Progesterone cream also is available over the counter. However, many of these products are ineffective because the progesterone content is too low, if present at all. Creams reported to contain adequate concentrations of progesterone include Pro-Gest, Bio Balance, and PhytoGest.[4] If these are too weak, a compounding pharmacy will need to prepare a stronger cream. Since the progesterone cream made by a compounding pharmacy is pharmaceutical grade and pure, I normally recommend it to my clients instead of the over-the-counter products.

A transdermal patch that combines estradiol with a synthetic progestin is now available at your local pharmacy. It is called CombiPatch, and it is applied in the same manner as an estrogen patch. However, the CombiPatch delivers two hormones directly into the bloodstream at once.

Vaginal and Rectal Routes

Although it sounds odd, compounding pharmacies can blend progesterone in water to create a rectal suspension. The user simply inserts a small syringe—with no needle—that has a special rectal tip and injects the medicine. It is rapidly absorbed, so leakage is not a problem. Sometimes bowel stimulation may occur, but this is not reported as often as with rectal suppositories.

Progesterone also can be molded into a wax base to form a suppository, which can be inserted vaginally or rectally. Suppositories are an effective means of delivering medication. However, when used vaginally, leakage—and sometimes irritation—can be a problem, and when used rectally, bowel stimulation can occur.

In an attempt to sidestep these annoyances, moistened progesterone capsules are another alternative for vaginal or rectal use. As with oral administration, multiple daily dosages normally are required for vaginal and rectal routes of administration of progesterone.

A vaginal gel of micronized progesterone (Crinone) is commercially available for use in assisted reproduction techniques. Currently, Wyeth-Ayerst, manufacturer of Premarin, is conducting clinical trials using Crinone for postmenopausal hormone replacement therapy.

Injections

As you can imagine, injections are not the method of choice for most women. Not only can injections be painful, but they also are inconvenient. However, this method is available, if needed.

Testosterone

"Testosterone! Isn't that a male hormone?" Many women are surprised to hear that they, too, produce small quantities of testosterone.

Testosterone falls under the classification of "male" hormones called androgens. Most of our androgens originate from our ovaries and adrenal glands, with an additional amount coming from fat tissue.

Androstenedione is a steroid precursor produced in the ovaries and adrenals that is converted into estrogen and testosterone. Women who transition through natural menopause may find that their androstenedione and testosterone levels decline gradually. Women who undergo a sudden menopause, however, become deficient in these hormones within 24 hours of surgery, as is the case with estrogen and progesterone levels.

Testosterone deficiency usually results in a flagging libido, changes in feelings of well-being, decreased bone density, and diminished muscle mass. Testosterone supplementation often is very effective, especially when used in combination with estrogen, for women who have undergone a sudden menopause. The trick is finding the proper dosage of the appropriate type of testosterone.

Women require far less testosterone than men do, so minute dosages go a long way. High dosages actually may make a woman feel worse and cause the frequently cited side effects of facial hair, acne, aggression, deepened voice, adverse lipid profile, and elevated liver enzymes. The degree of tolerance also may be influenced by the type of androgen prescribed: synthetic (for example, methyltestosterone) or "natural" (bio-identical micronized natural testosterone).

Synthetic preparations use types of testosterone that are slightly different chemically from what is produced by the body. These preparations are formulated in dosages that are too high for most women. For example, the most commonly prescribed oral estrogen-testosterone combination is Estratest. Full-strength Estratest contains 1.25 mg of esterified estrogens with 2.5 mg of methyltestosterone, and half-strength Estratest HS contains .625 mg of esterified estrogen with 1.25 mg of methyltestosterone. Many practitioners agree that most women require even less testosterone than is present in the half-strength version, yet that is what is commercially available and, therefore, what is prescribed.

Synthetic versions of testosterone, especially at these higher levels, can create unpleasant and harmful side effects. As with any combination product, individualized dosages cannot be made because of the fixed amounts of each medicine. However, compounding pharmacies can supply methyltestosterone in the lower dosage recommended by proponents of testosterone therapy, which is 0.25 mg to 0.75 mg of methyltestosterone per day.[5]

One advantage to using methyltestosterone is that it is not metabolized into estrogen as readily as its "natural" counterpart.[6] This could be beneficial to women who would like to enjoy the benefits of testosterone therapy with minimal elevation of estrogen levels. An example would be women with estrogen-dependent cancers.

"Natural" testosterone is not commercially available and needs to be obtained through a compounding pharmacy. Remember that the "natural" version of a hormone is so called because it is chemically manufactured to be identical to what is produced in the body. That's the attraction of natural testosterone. When compounded, natural testosterone can be prescribed in low dosages, combined with other hormones, and administered in a variety of ways. All of these benefits add up to a safer regimen, because the incidences of virilizing effects and liver interference are significantly lower.

Advantages of Testosterone

Sex Drive

A few months after her hysterectomy with BSO for large uterine fibroids, *JULIE*, a 41-year-old college professor, noticed that her sex drive had disappeared. Although the estrogen-testosterone combination Estratest HS (half strength) improved her libido, it triggered headaches and acne. Conflicted about her options, she scheduled an appointment with me. I gave her information on natural testosterone and suggested that she talk to her nurse practitioner about it. Julie's nurse practitioner was in agreement and worked closely with a compounding pharmacist to determine a dosage that would fuel Julie's sex drive without inducing side effects. Whether due to the lower dosage of testosterone, the natural estrogen and testosterone, or both, Julie was satisfied with her new HRT regimen.

When a woman notes that her sex drive has plummeted, it usually is at the top of her list of concerns, yet she may be reluctant to bring up the subject. For that reason, I bring up the topic whenever I teach a class or provide health counseling. Once the floodgate has been opened, I am usually inundated with questions.

Often, women do not even realize that the changes in their sex drives are related to sudden menopause. They usually are relieved to discover that there "isn't something else wrong" with them.

Testosterone therapy usually is quite effective at restoring a waning libido and also has the added benefit of relieving vaginal dryness, which is another barrier to intimacy. This is especially true when estrogen is included in the regimen, because estrogen "primes the pump," so to speak. Either used alone or in combination, testosterone should help to increase sexual desire.

Memory

Most studies examining the link between hormones and cognition focus on estrogen; however, some of them have included androgens. While many women report improvement of memory, concentration, and expressive language when estradiol levels are restored, others report just as much relief from the inclusion of testosterone. Whether testosterone's effects are independent of estrogen or the result of a collaborative relationship, it does appear to exert some influence on brain function.

Other Perks

Breast tenderness often is a side effect of estrogen or a progestational agent. Whether this is the result of a proliferation of breast tissue or from fluid retention, it can translate into slightly enlarged, painful breasts. If this is the case, it is advantageous that testosterone counteracts these effects by slightly reducing breast size.

Another perk to taking testosterone is that it may help replenish your vitality. Women who are hormone deficient often report a loss of energy and ambition. When testosterone levels are low and replacement therapy is initiated, many women find that they return to their "old selves." It is common for women to describe this as an increase in well-being.

Other ways that testosterone may help include maintaining muscle mass and strength and relieving hot flashes when estrogen alone does not do the trick.

Osteoporosis

It is well-established that estrogen plays an integral role in bone development, and in recent years, progesterone's pivotal role also has been showcased. But what about testosterone? Well, it appears that you can add this benefit to testosterone's list of virtues.

Testosterone helps to manufacture bone of superior quality and to preserve its density. In conjunction with calcium, it maintains bone mineralization. For example, two studies that were presented at the fifth annual meeting of the North American Menopause Society and reported in the *Journal of the American Medical*

Association in 1994 demonstrated that when testosterone was added to estrogen therapy, it stimulated bone formation and increased bone density.

The first study compared women taking conjugated equine estrogen (Premarin) with women taking esterified estrogen and methyltestosterone (Estratest) for 9 weeks. Both groups received 1,500 mg of calcium per day via dietary and supplemental sources. Then, three markers of bone breakdown found in urine and three markers of bone formation found in blood were measured. After treatment with estrogen alone (plus calcium), all markers of bone demineralization decreased by 15 percent to 40 percent. The women treated with the estrogen-androgen combination (plus calcium) also sustained a decrease in bone-loss markers, and additionally, their bone-formation markers either stabilized or increased by 10 percent to 15 percent.[7]

The second study involved 310 women who had undergone hysterectomies with BSO. After 6 months, the women on the estrogen-androgen combination enjoyed an increase in bone density. The author cautioned that these were preliminary findings, yet they were suggestive of a decrease in osteoporosis risk among these women.[8]

Disadvantages of Testosterone

Side Effects

Mention taking testosterone to most women and you are likely to hear, "I don't want a deep voice and a mustache." While it is true that side effects of testosterone treatment in women include acne, aggression, male-pattern hair growth, and virilization (deepening of the voice and enlargement of the clitoris), they are not common when testosterone is used in responsible doses. If these side effects do occur, lowering the dosage usually is helpful. If the medicine is discontinued, these changes are reversible.

Another frequently cited concern with testosterone usage is liver impairment. Again, the risk of this is low when supplementing with small amounts and by using "natural" testosterone.

If you have any form of liver disease or impairment, taking testosterone is not a good option for you. I believe that obtaining a serum lipid profile—which measures total cholesterol, HDL, LDL, and triglyceride levels—and liver enzymes annually is a prudent approach to monitoring the effects of testosterone therapy.

Methods of Administration

Of the three hormones available for postmenopausal hormone replacement therapy (estrogen, progesterone, and testosterone), testosterone is the least frequently prescribed. Much of what is known about androgens has been derived from studies designed for men.

I do not believe that this is a deliberate gender bias on the part of the researchers. It is just that for so long, testosterone's role in the development of women's bodies has not been addressed. Even today, many women do not realize that androgens exist outside of a man's body. This lack of direction is why many physicians feel uncomfortable prescribing testosterone for their female patients.

The good news for women who have had hysterectomies with BSO is that we are the ones most likely to receive testosterone. That is not to say that some of those who undergo natural menopause are not candidates for it, simply that doctors are more hesitant to use it with that patient population.

It is important to remember that if a woman's uterus is intact and she is taking estrogen as well as testosterone, she needs to be on a progestational agent to counteract the possibility of uterine cancer.

Oral

Oral testosterone comes in the form of capsules and sublingual tablets. The sublingual method allows the tablets to dissolve beneath the tongue, like nitroglycerine for heart patients. This method avoids the hepatic first-pass effect since it bypasses the digestive tract and enters the bloodstream directly.

If methyltestosterone is prescribed for postmenopausal HRT, it usually is in combination with an estrogen preparation. An example of this is Estratest, full or half strength, which is commercially available. Since this product comes in dosages higher than most women need, you should be closely monitored while using it.

If a woman wants to try testosterone therapy but has a history of an estrogen-linked tumor, methyltestosterone, which is not as readily converted to estrogen, alone can be initiated. Compounding pharmacies also offer methyltestosterone in lower amounts than what is commercially available. Suggested dosages range from 0.25 mg to 0.75 mg per day.

Micronized "natural" testosterone is available in capsule form and can be compounded alone or in combination with estrogen and progesterone. As with other compounded preparations, dosages are customized. However, a standard range for natural testosterone is 2 mg to 4 mg per day.

Transdermal

As with estrogen and progesterone, testosterone can be compounded into a cream or gel. It is then massaged into the skin of the torso, arms, or legs and enters directly into the bloodstream. Estrogen and progesterone can be added to the recipe if desired.

Currently a micronized testosterone patch is being tested. It is in the clinical trial phase; hopefully it will soon become available by prescription at your local pharmacy.

Vaginal/Genital Route

Topical application of testosterone cream to the clitoral area is helpful in combating genital atrophy that has not fully responded to vaginal estrogen cream. Some practitioners report that this also helps with urinary changes. Testosterone cream may be prescribed for use daily until the genital tissue becomes supple and responsive, at which time the medication is usually tapered off to a few times per week. If clitoromegaly (enlarged clitoris) occurs, the cream should be discontinued. In addition to its localized effects, some of the medication is absorbed into the system, so it improves sex drive.

Another option to the cream is the vaginal suppository. The effects of this method are comparable to those of the cream, providing an alternative for the treatment of vaginal symptoms. As with most genital hormonal preparations, some women find them messy to use.

Injections

Injections are not commonly used for postmenopausal HRT, mainly because there are other, more convenient and appealing methods of obtaining testosterone. However, some physicians utilize injections in women who are having difficulty maintaining adequate testosterone levels.

"How Long Should I Take Hormones?"

"The hormones have really helped my symptoms, but how long should I take them?" This was the question from *FRAN*, a 42-year-old secretary. Fran entered sudden menopause after she underwent a hysterectomy with BSO for a prolapsed uterus. She did not want to "monkey around" with supplements or soy products, so she went directly to hormones. She did not have any adjustment problems and felt "great." However, she was wondering if there was a specific period of time that she should remain on the hormones. Since she was using them for symptomatic relief, she and her doctor decided that she should stay on them until about age 50—the average age of a natural menopause.

Once you have hit upon the right combination or recipe of hormones for you, you will begin to feel much better. The menopausal changes you were experiencing should at least improve, if not disappear. Because most women who undergo sudden menopause do so as a result of a hysterectomy with BSO, they generally remain on HRT for several years. Although there is no specific period of time that a sudden menopausal woman (or any other woman, for that matter) should remain on HRT, the younger she is at the time of menopause, the longer she usually stays on it. This is for symptom management as well as for the prevention of osteoporosis and heart disease. If breast cancer is a threat, however, HRT may be used for only a few years to ease the shock to the body brought on by a sudden menopause. Then, other steps can be taken to alleviate symptoms, and medications can be used to prevent osteoporosis, if needed. Otherwise, a woman usually stays on HRT until she reaches the age of natural menopause, at which time the decision is reevaluated.

Not only does HRT assist in dealing with the physical and emotional changes of menopause, but it also confers protection to the bones, heart, brain, and colon for as long as you take the medication. If these issues are your primary concern, you may choose to remain on HRT indefinitely. However, some women want to remain on HRT only on a short-term basis to ease the shock to their bodies caused by sudden menopause. Others simply change their minds about the decision to use HRT.

Some sudden menopausal women may opt to discontinue HRT at about the age of natural menopause (45 to 55 years). If this is the case, do not discontinue your medicine "cold turkey," or you may promptly begin having severe problems once again. Instead, wean yourself off of the hormones gradually, tapering the number of days per week that you use the medication or decreasing the dosage. This usually is accomplished over a period of a few months. Your health-care practitioner can provide you with direction.

If the menopausal changes that drove you to initiate HRT resume, you can then evaluate whether you want to continue taking the medicine or try using complementary therapies.

Reference Tables

The five tables that start on page 163 provide convenient summaries of the information contained in this chapter. Additionally, they include more detailed information about dosages available and typical regimens.

One Final Thought

After reading this chapter, I think you can understand how prescribing HRT is both a science and an art. It may take several months of adjustments before you feel close to your "old self" again. Sometimes all of the choices available for postmenopausal HRT are overwhelming, but I truly believe this is a benefit. It means that more alternatives exist to restore the hormonal balance to your body.

I also believe that if all women underwent routine checks of their hormone levels starting at about age 30 (or prior to a hysterectomy or to anticipated ovarian failure in younger women), it would take much of the guesswork out of HRT. At least then women and their health-care providers would have baseline comparisons available when determining the appropriate dosages of hormones.

More clinicians are using saliva testing rather then blood testing for the quantitative analysis of "free" hormone levels. Free hormones are those that are not bound to proteins in the blood and, therefore, are available to bind with the hormone receptors throughout the body to quell the menopausal changes. They are the biologically active hormones that are detectable in the saliva. It is a simple, painless, noninvasive test that can be performed at home with the specimen transported to a lab through the mail. It also is possible to detect free-hormone levels in the blood, if specifically ordered.

Whether you choose to use HRT, complementary therapies, or both to help ease the changes associated with menopause, it is encouraging to know that options exist and that researchers are continually looking at new and improved methods of treatment. Not very long ago, women facing these issues had only one course of action—to resign themselves to the changes and move on.

Table 6.1: Examples of Commercially Available Hormone Replacement Therapy Products

ESTROGEN

Oral

Estradiol (Estrace), 0.5 mg, 1 mg, 2 mg

Conjugated equine estrogens, primarily estrone (Premarin), 0.3 mg, 0.625 mg, 0.9 mg, 1.25 mg, 2.5 mg

Conjugated estrogens (Cenestin), 0.625 mg, 0.9 mg, 1.25 mg

Estropipate, estrone (Ogen, Ortho-Est), 0.625 mg, 1.25 mg, 2.5 mg

Esterified estrogen (Estratab and Menest), 0.3 mg, 0.625 mg, 1.25 mg, 2.5 mg

Oral combined

Conjugated equine estrogens with medroxyprogesterone acetate (Premphase cyclic: Premarin and Cycrin), 0.625 mg/5 mg

Conjugated equine estrogens with medroxyprogesterone acetate (Prempro continuous: Premarin and Cycrin), 0.625mg/2.5 mg, 0.625 mg/5 mg

Norethindrone acetate/ethinyl estradiol (femhrt), 1 mg/5 mcg

Esterified estrogen with methyltestosterone (Estratest HS/Estratest), 0.625 mg/1.25 mg, 1.25 mg/2.5 mg

Estradiol with norgestimate (Ortho-Prefest), 1 mg/0.09 mg

Transdermal

Estradiol patch: Estraderm (0.05 mg, 0.1 mg); Climara (0.025 mg, 0.05 mg, 0.075 mg, 0.1 mg); Vivelle (0.0375 mg, 0.05 mg, 0.075 mg, 0.1 mg); FemPatch (0.025 mg); Alora (0.05 mg, 0.075 mg, 0.1 mg)

Estradiol with norethindrone acetate patch: CombiPatch (0.05 mg/0.14 mg, 0.05 mg/0.25 mg)

Vaginal cream

Estrogen vaginal cream, dosages vary: Estrace (0.1 mg/g), Premarin (0.625 mg/g), Ogen (1.5 mg/g), Dienestrol (0.1 mg/g)

Vaginal ring

Estradiol vaginal ring (Estring), 2 mg

Table 6.1: Examples of Commercially Available Hormone Replacement Therapy Products (cont'd.)

PROGESTERONE/PROGESTINS

Oral

Micronized progesterone (Prometrium), 100 mg, 200 mg

Medroxyprogesterone acetate (Provera, Cycrin, Amen, Curretab), 2.5 mg, 5 mg, 10 mg

Megestrol acetate (Megace), 20 mg, 40 mg

Norethindrone acetate (Aygestin), 5 mg

Oral combined

Conjugated equine estrogens with medroxyprogesterone acetate (Premphase cyclic: Premarin and Cycrin), 0.625 mg/5 mg

Conjugated equine estrogens with medroxyprogesterone acetate (Prempro continuous: Premarin and Cycrin), 0.625mg/2.5 mg, 0.625 mg/5 mg

Estradiol with norgestimate (Ortho-Prefest), 1 mg/0.09 mg

Norethindrone acetate/ethinyl estradiol (femhrt), 1 mg/5 mcg

Transdermal

Estradiol with norethindrone acetate patch: CombiPatch (0.05 mg/0.14 mg, 0.05 mg/0.25 mg)

TESTOSTERONE*

Oral

Fluoxymesterone (Halotestin), 2 mg, 5 mg, 10 mg

Oral combined

Esterified estrogen with methyltestosterone (Estratest HS/ Estratest), 0.625 mg/1.25 mg, 1.25 mg/2.5 mg

*None of the testosterone preparations commercially available are the micronized, "natural" testosterone. Contact a compounding pharmacy for this type of testosterone preparation.

Table 6.2: Possible Side Effects of Hormone Replacement Therapy

ESTROGENS

Fluid retention/bloating

Breast changes (tenderness, enlargement, secretions)

Weight gain

Headaches

Nausea

PROGESTINS/PROGESTERONES

Fluid retention/bloating

Breast changes (tenderness, enlargement, secretions)

Weight gain

Headaches

PMS-like symptoms

Irritability

Depression

Nausea

TESTOSTERONE

Acne/oily skin

Decreased breast size

Increased facial and body hair

Irritability/aggression

Nausea

Table 6.3: Contraindications for Use of Hormone Replacement Therapy

ABSOLUTE

Estrogen-dependent tumors, particularly breast and endometrial

Undiagnosed, abnormal uterine bleeding

Liver impairment*

Active thrombophlebitis or thromboembolic disorders, especially if associated with previous estrogen use

*Transdermal/vaginal routes may be considered.

QUESTIONABLE

History of breast or reproductive cancers

History of stroke, cardiovascular disease, deep vein thrombosis, liver disease*

Gallbladder disease*

Cigarette smoking

Migraine headaches*

Asthma

*Transdermal/vaginal routes may be considered.

Table 6.4: Suggested Supplemental Postmenopausal Hormone Ranges

	SERUM (BLOOD)	SALIVA
Estradiol	100 ng/dl–200 ng/dl	0.5 pg/ml–5.0 pg/ml
Progesterone	5 ng/dl–15 ng/dl	.05 pg/ml–0.5 pg/ml
Testosterone	30 ng/dl–50 ng/dl	20 pg/ml–50 pg/ml
	*nanograms per deciliter	*picograms per milliliter

These serum figures represent suggested guidelines for total hormone levels, not "free" (active) hormone levels. Saliva and serum parameters vary according to the laboratory used.

Source: Women's Health Access Newsletter, Women's Health America Group

Table 6.5: Sample Hormone Replacement Therapy Regimens

	ESTROGEN	PROGESTA-TIONAL AGENT	WITHDRAWAL BLEEDING
Post-hysterectomy continuous	Daily	May or may not be used	None
Cyclic sequential	21–25 days/month	7–12 days concomitant with estrogen	During the 5–7 days not on medicine
Continuous sequential	Daily	First or last 12–14 days/month	After the last day of progesta-tional agent
Cyclic combined	21–25 days/month	21–25 days/month concomitant with estrogen	During the 5–7 days not on medicine
Continuous combined	Daily	Daily	Irregular bleed-ing during the first year, then usually amenor-rheic

Chapter Highlights

▣ The decision to try HRT should be based on the need for symptomatic relief of sudden menopausal changes, as well as for protection from long-term health issues such as osteoporosis and heart disease. The role of your personal and family medical history of cancer, osteoporosis, and heart disease should weigh heavily in your decision.

▣ Hysterectomized women do not require progesterone, but may opt to use it with estrogen and testosterone. A woman with an intact uterus who has undergone a sudden menopause does need progesterone in her hormonal cocktail to protect her from uterine cancer.

▣ When using HRT, start off with the "natural" (bio-identical) versions of estrogen, progesterone, and testosterone. These can be found at your local pharmacy or through a compounding pharmacy. The exception is testosterone, which must be prepared by a compounding pharmacy. If you have a past history of an estrogen-dependent cancer and are opting to try testosterone, you may want to use a low dosage of the synthetic form (methyltestosterone). Methyltestosterone is not as readily converted to estrogen as is the micronized, natural form.

▣ Remember that prescribing HRT is not an exact science. Every woman is different, and therefore some trial and error may need to occur. Your needs may also change as you age, and your HRT may need to be adjusted accordingly.

Doc Talk

▣ Before beginning HRT, be sure to have a mammogram, Pap smear and pelvic exam, lipid profile, and bone-density test. When using testosterone, add liver enzymes to the list of tests, and be sure to have them and your lipid profile checked annually while taking testosterone. If you have a

history of cancer, discuss with your doctor the need for
additional screening tests.

- Talk to your doctor about finding out your baseline hormone
  levels before initiating HRT. Even though these levels are apt
  to be low in a sudden menopausal woman, this baseline will
  help to interpret hormone levels after HRT has been started.
  Give consideration to checking saliva levels rather than
  serum levels, since saliva is more convenient and accurate.
  If your doctor is checking your blood levels, ask whether
  testing for "free" (active) hormone levels is available at
  the lab.

- In the past, women who had breast cancer were
  automatically excluded from using HRT. However, some
  doctors are prescribing it in a select group of breast cancer
  survivors. If you are contemplating HRT and you had an
  early-stage breast tumor that had no lymph node
  involvement and that was not estrogen dependent, and if
  you also have been cancer free for at least 2 years, discuss
  your options with your doctor. Some physicians are using
  HRT under the same circumstances in women who had
  estrogen-dependent tumors but who have been cancer free
  for at least 5 years.

- Be sure to keep your doctor informed about whether the
  hormones prescribed are alleviating your menopausal
  symptoms, as well as about any side effects. Your doctor
  may need to adjust your dosage or try different forms of the
  hormones to find the "recipe" that is best for you.

- Whether or not you opt for HRT, reevaluate your decision
  annually. Take into consideration any changes in your health
  status as well as any new information on hormones.

7

Creating Health

One January 1, a friend of mine, *EMILY*, made a New Year's resolution to adopt a healthier lifestyle. At the time, she was a 50-year-old psychologist in a very busy practice. Due to the nature of her work, she was sedentary most of the day. She was slightly overweight, did not get any regular exercise, and had a chronic health problem that was well controlled. Since her aging parents lived with her, she was their sole caretaker and assumed both physical and financial responsibility for them.

After working all day and caring for her parents, Emily did not maintain much of a social life. As a result of all this, she did not feel good about herself physically or emotionally. She was tired, lacked energy, and was rather unhappy about the direction in which her life was going. She recognized that this was an unhealthy way to live, hence her New Year's resolution.

However, long before the end of the year, guess what happened? Nothing. Emily was still stuck in the same old rut. I think we all can relate to that. Just think of the countless New Year's resolutions that have come and gone unfulfilled. Our intentions are good, but change is easier said than done.

When Emily initially decided to turn her life around, she asked for my help. Together we mapped out a new dietary approach, as well as some plans for incorporating exercise into her schedule while still giving her time for a bit of relaxation. Periodically, I would call and invite her places to get her out of the house and socialize. However, she always had an excuse for why she could not implement any of the strategies.

After 6 months of this, it finally dawned on me that I was doing all of the work here. Emily said she wanted to change, but I was the one putting forth all of the effort. That would be a pretty good deal if it actually worked! That's when I realized that only she had the capability of creating health in her life. I could not do it for her. All of my good intentions were for naught. I could give her the tools to take her life in a new direction, but she had to do the work.

———

That's really the moral of my story. We all have the potential to change and improve our lives, but the change has to come from within. No one can do it for you.

To me, health is more than merely the absence of illness. Just because you are not sick does not mean that you are healthy.

What's your definition of health? Have you ever given it much thought? My definition of health is the achievement of a state of harmony between body, mind, and spirit.

A large part of this is your own desire to participate in maintaining your physical, emotional, and spiritual well-being. The basic premise is that health does not just happen to you. It is not something that is bestowed upon you. It is an active, dynamic process over which you have influence. Sure, there are some factors over which we have no control, but we can influence the vast majority of factors. Instead of fixating on those we cannot influence, doesn't it make sense to focus on those we can?

I am convinced that every action we take and every thought we have impacts our immune response. Anything that affects body, mind, or spirit has the ability to influence the integrity of the immune system. Once the immune system is impaired, it becomes vulnerable to bacteria and viruses, as well as to cancer-causing agents (carcinogens).

When it comes to boosting immunity, I believe that it boils down to making sound lifestyle choices on a daily basis. For example, how many hours of sleep did you get last night? Did you skip breakfast this morning, or did you fuel your body with a balanced meal? Do you suffer from stress-related ailments?

If, as you are reading this, you are answering the questions in dismay and thinking, "Boy, I have a lot of room for improvement," do not despair. It is entirely possible to turn your life around by developing a new "life plan."

Simply admitting that you need to make some changes is half the battle. The other half is sticking with your plan until it becomes ingrained as a normal part of your life. This chapter is designed to provide you with a launchpad to skyrocket you to better health and well-being.

Ten Tips for Creating Health

1. Trace Your Family Health Tree

Have you ever been told that you have your father's eyes or your mother's facial shape or your grandmother's hair? Relatives often make those comments about the traits they have passed along in their genes, but how often do you hear them remarking on your family health tree? It is just as likely that you share their risk for certain diseases, such as hypertension, diabetes, or cancer.

I think we all can acknowledge the importance of knowing our family history, but how many of us take the time to research it and put it on paper? In fact, it is rather simple to do. It is basically a written record of your relatives and any illnesses or diseases they've had, along with their causes of death.

This is crucial information that helps to determine your predisposition for a particular disorder. This information often is referred to as knowing what "runs in your family." Having a disease that runs in your family does not necessarily mean that you will develop the problem, but being aware of your family history will help you and your doctor evaluate your risk for certain diseases.

One of the most tragic public examples of being unaware of the role of family history can be seen in Gilda Radner's situation. Gilda was a regular cast member of the comedy show "Saturday Night Live" in the seventies. In 1989, she died of ovarian cancer after battling the disease for 2½ years. She was diagnosed with late-stage cancer in 1986 after 10 months of traveling across the country from specialist to specialist and undergoing numerous medical tests in an attempt to establish a reason for her symptoms.

Because ovarian cancer is an insidious disease, it is difficult to diagnose in the early stages. It wasn't until Gilda shared the news of her cancer with her family that she and her doctor discovered that she had numerous close relatives with breast and ovarian cancer. Because of her genetic tree, her risk of ovarian cancer skyrocketed. I cannot help but wonder what might have happened if her doctors had had this information early on, when she began having symptoms.

As this sad story demonstrates, one of the greatest gifts you can give posterity is a documented family health tree. Ultimately, it can help save your life, as well as ensure you a high quality of life.

The benefits of recording your medical pedigree are plentiful. For example, it will influence the frequency and type of health screenings you get (which can aid in early detection), it can motivate you to kick some of your unhealthy habits (prevention), and it will serve as a valuable tool as scientists continue to locate the genes that cause more than 2,000 hereditary illnesses.

There are many ways to unearth this information about your family health history. If you wish to be systematic and methodical, consult some of the books and articles that have been written on the subject. They will guide you step-by-step through the process.

However, I do not think your effort must be that exhaustive. Getting started simply entails mapping out your family tree and talking to your relatives.

Be aware that this may be a sensitive issue for some of them. Some people are reluctant to disclose personal information. They consider it an invasion of their privacy and may not want to reopen old wounds. It may put them at ease if you explain that your intention is not to be nosy but to protect your family from unnecessary pain and suffering.

On the other hand, you are likely to run across relatives who do nothing but talk about their medical problems. They can actually be a blessing in disguise, because they are a wellspring of information.

The further back you delve into your heritage, the more difficult accessing information becomes. Elderly relatives and friends of your deceased relatives may possess valuable knowledge but have trouble recalling it. Instead of asking them specific medical questions about a person, get them to describe the person's life—likes and dislikes, personality, milestones, etc. Often by reminiscing, they begin to remember important details that otherwise would elude them. You also can check with the local vital-records bureau for cause of death, listed on the death certificate.

As you are gathering your family data, you may notice that it is peppered with numerous diseases and become alarmed. Keep in mind that it is a pattern of illness that is of particular importance, especially if the age of onset seems rather young; for example, a heart attack at age 40.

People sometimes tend to focus on the "heavy hitter" diseases such as heart attack, stroke, and cancer, while overlooking other equally notable problems. Examples of these include allergies, diabetes, asthma, mental illness, depression, eating disorders, birth defects, miscarriages, multiple sclerosis, osteoporosis, anemia, alcoholism, and substance abuse.

The easiest way to keep track of this information on your health tree is to make a key in the corner of the chart and assign an abbreviation to each disorder. Then, beneath each person's name, concisely record the particular illness, age of onset, and age of death.

Once you have actually diagrammed your genealogical health tree, the second step is sharing this information with your doctor. This will help the two of you evaluate your risk for diseases, interpret any symptomatology you may develop, and determine if these problems are predominantly rooted in genetics, lifestyle habits, or a combination of both factors. Genetic counseling also may be advisable.

To help you get started on your quest toward prevention and early detection, I have included a table of screening exams to use as a guideline for determining what you need and when you need it.

The calendar on the next page represents a sample of health maintenance guidelines for healthy individuals without symptoms. It is not a comprehensive table, nor is it intended to be a substitute for medical advice. Consult your physician to develop a schedule that meets your individual needs.

Sources: American Cancer Society; American College of Obstetrics and Gynecology; Guide to Clinical Preventive Services, second edition, U.S. Preventive Services Task Force, 1996; National Cancer Institute.

2. Kick Your Unhealthy Habits

Breaking your unhealthy habits falls into the category of taking responsibility for your choices. Virtually every aspect of our lives is in some way malleable. Maybe something cannot be completely changed, but perhaps a certain part of it can be changed.

Think of the free will involved in making decisions regarding eating, exercising, smoking, managing stress, improving relationships, and choosing a job. Sometimes being reminded that these are choices that we make is the catalyst for examining the quality of our lives. Do you like who you are and where you are in your life? If not, what can you do about it?

Many times, when I counsel people on modifying their lifestyles, they look at me as if I'm crazy. This is usually followed by creative excuses for why the suggestions I outlined couldn't possibly work for them. Sometimes they even say things like, "You've got to be kidding" or "You want me to do what?" or "I thought I would come in here and you would just tell me which vitamins to take so I'll feel better. Isn't there an easier way?"

Table 7.1: Schedule of Screening Exams

Type of examination	Age: 20s and 30s	Age: 40s and 50s	Age: 60+
Physical exam/ medical history	Every 1–3 years	Every 1–3 years	Every 1–3 years
Blood pressure	Every visit to the doctor, 1–3 years	Every visit to the doctor, 1–3 years	Every visit to the doctor, 1–3 years
Cholesterol	Every 5 years	Every 5 years	Every 5 years
Breast self-exam	Monthly	Monthly	Monthly
Breast exam by doctor	Yearly	Yearly	Yearly
Mammogram	Baseline at 40	Every 1–2 years during 40s, yearly during 50s	Yearly
Pap smear/pelvic exam	Yearly	Yearly	Yearly
Skin check (self)	Monthly	Monthly	Monthly
Rectal exam (digital/stool test)	None	Yearly	Yearly
Rectal exam (colonoscopy)	None	Baseline at 50, every 3–5 years	Every 3–5 years
Vision	None	Every 2–4 years	Every 1–2 years
Hearing	None	Every 3 years	Every 3 years, yearly at 65
Tetanus/diphtheria	Every 10 years	Every 10 years	Every 10 years
Influenza vaccine (flu shot)	None	None	Yearly at 65
Pneumonia vaccine	None	None	Once at 65 or older
Dental exam	Every 6 mths –1 year	Every 6 mths –1 year	Every 6 mths –1 year

I usually reply that I didn't say it was going to be easy. After all, for the most part, strange diseases are not killing us. Our lifestyles are killing us. And we have a lot of control over that, don't we?

The Journal of the American Medical Association published a study showing that half of all deaths are attributed to 10 factors that are rooted in lifestyle, deeming those deaths premature. The factors include the following:[1]

- Smoking—Smoking is directly related to 30 percent of all cancer deaths and 21 percent of all cardiovascular deaths.

- High-fat diet—The combination of a high-fat diet and lack of regular exercise is linked to 14 percent of all deaths.

- Lack of regular exercise.

- Drinking and driving—Alcohol is a factor in 40 to 50 percent of all car accidents.

- Failure to keep immunizations up to date—Adult vaccines include tetanus, diphtheria, flu, pneumonia, and hepatitis.

- Toxic substances at work and at home—These include asbestos, secondhand smoke, pesticides, radon, and lead.

- Failure to keep firearms under lock and key.

- Sexual promiscuity—Sexually transmitted diseases cause 30,000 deaths per year and are among the fastest growing causes of death.

- Failure to wear a seatbelt, and speeding.

- Drug and alcohol abuse.

At first glance, you might be tempted to think this top-10 list is rather discouraging, but I find it encouraging—because we have the ability to alter these factors. These are preventable causes of death. For the most part, these factors represent choices we make. But knowing that, we then must decide to change our harmful habits. The catch is, in many cases, we have been doing these things for so long it might seem easier to continue than to change.

Thirty-nine-year-old STEPHANIE is a perfect example of recognizing unhealthy habits and desiring to change them. I met Stephanie when she went through a Heart Check screening program at the Hamot Health Connection, a women's center where I work as a health counselor and educator. Heart Check is designed to determine a person's risk for heart attack.

Stephanie went from station to station where she had her height, weight, blood pressure, and cholesterol screened, and she completed a cardiac risk-appraisal survey. A computer analyzed the data, made suggestions for improvement related to each risk factor, and calculated her chances of suffering a heart attack. Stephanie received her results and they were not good. Her blood pressure, cholesterol, and weight were significantly elevated. Without modifying her lifestyle, she was headed for a heart attack.

Since the results of the Heart Check scared her, Stephanie scheduled an appointment to discuss them with me. I spent an hour providing encouragement and guidance, and together we outlined a life plan that would lead to better health.

You can probably imagine how overwhelming it was for her as she realized the magnitude of the changes she needed to make. I even caught a glimpse of self-doubt in her eyes. I suggested she start working on one or two areas at a time, instead of trying to change everything at once. This would make things more manageable for her. The idea of incremental changes seemed to buoy her self-confidence. She realized that she had some tough changes to make, but stated that her life was worth it.

In contrast with Stephanie's attitude, I recall a conversation with another patient who was equally overwhelmed about the lifestyle changes needed to bring her cardiac risk profile into safe ranges. At the end of our visit, she said to me, "Isn't alcohol good for your heart?" I knew where she was going with this and replied, "Yes, it can help to lower your cholesterol level." "Well, don't you worry about me, dear," she said. "I love wine and I'll just have a glass with dinner every night."

This was her solution. Of course, a daily glass of wine could not possibly counteract the harmful effects of all her other risk factors, and I explained this to her. Change is more complex than drinking a glass of wine every day at dinner—and at first it may seem far less enjoyable. However, nothing makes you feel better than beginning to see the results of healthy new habits: quitting smoking, for example, and two weeks later realizing that for the first time in years you just climbed the stairs without feeling winded. Or one day noticing a shapely new muscle beneath your skin, developed during your month-old exercise routine. Pat yourself on the back for these achievements—don't discount even the seemingly "small" ones—and don't forget to be patient with yourself. Change and the building of new habits take time.

In the end it boils down to personal accountability. When we finally understand that a "life plan" is a process, not merely an event that we engage in for a short period of time, success will not be far behind. It is similar to the difference between running a marathon and running a sprint. Running a marathon is a commitment.

3. You Are What You Eat

"I know I don't eat well. Do you think that's why I'm tired and run down?" asked 37-year-old *LINDSAY*. For Lindsay, a typical day of eating consisted of skipping breakfast, chasing down a small bag of M&M's with a Diet Coke midmorning, eating a sandwich and fries for lunch, and finishing the day by ordering takeout for supper.

Lindsay knew that she needed to modify her diet, but she didn't realize the degree to which food influenced the way she felt and performed. To improve her knowledge of nutrition, I recommended nutrition counseling and cooking classes.

Most people think of food solely in terms of pleasure—what looks and tastes good. Of course, there is and should be a joyful aspect to eating. Who doesn't like to savor delicious tastes, ogle delectable morsels, and relish the wonderful aromas of our favorite foods? Yet there is a critical purpose of eating that we often forget: eating nourishes every cell in our bodies.

In order to optimize health and well-being, it is essential that we provide the body with the fuel it needs. For example, when you sit down to a meal of prime rib, French fries, and a beer, your mind might be thinking, "All right! I can't wait to take a bite of that mouth-watering steak, eat a few crispy fries, and then wash it all down with a cold beer."

But do you know what your body might be saying at the same time? "Aah, not again! I'd better gear up because I'm about to work overtime—from my digestive tract to my cardiovascular network to my immune system. And to make matters worse, at the end of this meal, she'll feel full, but I'll actually be starved because I will still be deprived of the nutrients I need to function."

Now, you might be thinking, "If only my body talked to me like this, I might make better choices." Believe it or not, your body does communicate this information to you. It communicates through your energy level, stamina, resistance to illness, feelings of well-being, quality of sleep, weight, cholesterol level, blood pressure—get the picture?

I am not suggesting that we have to turn our diets into science projects or that a piece of steak can never again pass our lips. We just need to maintain a sense of balance when it comes to our eating patterns and reestablish some sensible priorities, based on important nutritional principles.

If these principles have slipped your mind or if you never really knew them, turn to the Food Guide Pyramid for guidance. The Food Guide Pyramid is an illustration of guidelines for the number of daily servings you should consume from each of the major food groups.

Food Guide Pyramid

A Guide to Daily Food Choices

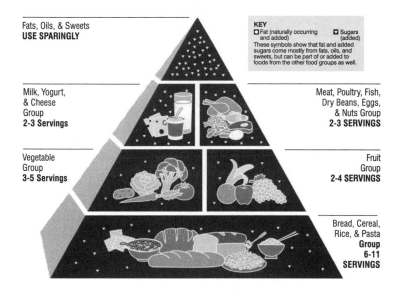

Figure 7.1: The Food Guide Pyramid

Source: U.S. Department of Agriculture and U.S. Department of Health and Human Services

---

A very simple principle of healthy eating is to consume the bulk of your calories during the day. Approximately ¾ of the calories your body burns off are done so by suppertime, unless you work second or third shift. Do you remember the old saying: eat breakfast like a queen, lunch like a princess, and supper like a pauper? It turns out there is some merit to that advice. Our calorie consumption should be like an inverted triangle, with a hearty breakfast, modest lunch, small dinner, and a few snacks in between. In reality, however, most of us do just the opposite. We skip breakfast, grab a quick lunch, and then eat almost continuously beginning with dinner. Our metabolisms may be slowing down in the evenings, but our mouths are not. This behavior results in unwanted pounds, not only from late-night eating but also from eating little or no breakfast. In fact, the body's metabolism is like a wood-burning stove. The embers die down at night, and in order to get it going again in the morning, it needs to be stoked. That is what breakfast does for the body; it stokes the metabolism.

Another important aspect of metabolism is muscle mass. Did you know that muscle tissue burns more calories than fat does? That's another benefit to exercising. Muscle may weigh more (which is why exercising is not always immediately reflected in the numbers on the scale), but you will lose inches as you become more toned, and you will boost your basal metabolic rate (the number of calories you burn at rest).

Let's not forget water's role in metabolism. Adult body weight is 55 percent to 65 percent water. Besides being necessary for fluid and electrolyte balance, nutrient delivery, waste removal, acid–base balance, and bodily fluid stability, water is needed to efficiently burn calories. It is recommended that individuals drink at least eight 8-ounce glasses of water per day.

These are just a few of the ABCs of nutrition. There are several other ways of improving health through diet and supplements. To help you get started, I've summarized information on five hot nutrition topics.

Strive for Five

The single best dietary action you can take to fortify your immune system is to eat a variety of fruits and vegetables. If you take a moment to examine the Food Guide Pyramid, you will note that the daily recommendations for fruits and vegetables are two to four and three to five servings respectively.

Unfortunately, most people do not follow these guidelines. In fact, it is estimated that only 9 percent of the population get the required minimum of five servings of fruits and vegetables daily.

When I perform health counseling, I do a cursory dietary assessment of my clients. One of the questions I ask my clients is how they are doing on fruits and vegetables. Do you get enough?

Table 7.2: What Counts as a Serving?

Bread, cereal, rice, and pasta group	1 slice bread 1 tortilla ½ cup cooked rice, pasta, or cereal 1 ounce ready-to-eat cereal ½ hamburger roll, bagel, or English muffin 3–4 plain crackers (small) 1 pancake (4-inch) ½ croissant (large) ½ doughnut or Danish (medium) ¹⁄₁₆ cake (average) 2 cookies (medium) ¹⁄₁₂ pie (2-crust, 8-inch)
Vegetable group	½ cup chopped raw or cooked vegetables 1 cup raw, leafy vegetables ¾ cup vegetable juice ½ cup scalloped potatoes ½ cup potato salad 10 French fries
Fruit group	1 piece fruit or melon wedge ¾ cup fruit juice ½ cup chopped, cooked, or canned fruit ¼ cup dried fruit
Milk, yogurt, and cheese group	1 cup milk or yogurt 1½ ounces natural cheese 2 ounces processed cheese 2 cups cottage cheese 1½ cups ice cream or ice milk 1 cup frozen yogurt
Meat, poultry, fish, dried beans, eggs, and nuts group	2½ to 3 ounces cooked lean beef, pork, lamb, veal, poultry, or fish (count ½ cup cooked beans or 1 egg or 2 tablespoons peanut butter or ⅓ cup nuts as 1 ounce of meat)
Fats, oils, and sweets	Use sparingly

Table 7.3: Lean Meat Choices

Beef	round tip
	top round
	eye of round
	top loin
	tenderloin
	sirloin
Pork	tenderloin
	boneless top loin chop
	boneless ham, cured
	center loin chop
Lamb	loin chop
	leg
Veal	cutlet
	loin chop

Source: U.S. Department of Agriculture and U.S. Department of Health and Human Services

Invariably they respond by saying yes. I then ask if they get at least five servings a day, to which they usually reply, "Five! Am I supposed to be getting that many?"

Most people report getting approximately three servings of fruits and vegetables a day. To help them work their way up to at least five servings, I suggest they add one more serving to their current intake. As soon as they have habitually incorporated that intake into their daily diets, they can continue to increase incrementally.

Upon discussing the issue of "striving for five," my clients tend to ask two questions: "How?" and "Why?" Let's start with why.

Often, people are in search of the "magic bullet" that will make them feel great and ward off illness. Generally, they are wistfully looking toward a particular vitamin or herb. In my opinion, fruits and vegetables come close. They are chock full of antioxidants and phytochemicals, both substances that neutralize the harmful oxidative processes that occur at the cellular level and trigger disease.

According to researcher Bruce N. Ames, Ph.D., and his colleagues at the University of California, Berkeley, people who neglect eating the minimum requirement of five servings of antioxidant-laden foods—including fruits, vegetables, and whole grains—sustain twice the risk of developing cancer as people who get enough of these foods.[2]

Additionally, these food sources are rich in fiber and very low in fat. Not only does fiber increase satiety—and therefore you are likely to eat less food—but it also helps lower the risk of heart disease as well as of certain cancers. Current recommendations suggest that individuals eat 25 to 35 grams of fiber daily. It is best to increase your intake of fiber gradually to lower the chances of bloating.

Let's not forget another important reason to eat fruits and vegetables—they taste good!

As to the question of how to get five servings of fruits and vegetables daily, that takes a little thought and planning. Try experimenting and becoming creative with your choices. However, if your idea of fruit is a glass of juice and a vegetable is a plate of mashed potatoes, it may take you a while longer to widen your horizons.

Take some time to go to the farmer's market or the grocery store and look around at all of the produce. The variety and selection are fabulous. You are bound to find fruits and vegetables to your liking.

Once you get them home and get your kitchen stocked with good fruits and vegetables, that's half the battle. You now have them available to eat. You just have to remember to include them in your meals and snacks. Keep in mind that frozen and canned fruits and vegetables are nutritious and can be a time saver, as can dried fruit. For you gardeners, there is nothing quite like eating the fruits of your own labor. If you freeze or can your homegrown produce, you will enjoy it year round.

One last note about fresh fruits and vegetables: before you enjoy eating them, be sure to wash them. This helps to remove dirt and pesticide residue. I like to wash the produce as soon as I get it home so that I don't forget. Washing it in advance also saves time later on when I may be rushed and less inclined to eat them if I have to stop and wash them first.

As a safety precaution, you may wish to eat only locally grown, seasonal fruits and vegetables if possible. If the item of your choice is not in season locally, inquire at the market as to the item's origins. Other countries may not have the same food regulations for quality control and pesticide usage as the United States. Although all imported produce is supposed to be spot checked when it enters the country, these practices and methods have come under question recently.

The Joy of Soy

A 42-year-old nurse friend of mine who entered sudden menopause asked me what she could do about her hot flashes and night sweats. After I listed some of the coping strategies and lifestyle changes she could make, I asked her if she would consider using soy products. She replied, "Oh no, I like regular milk too much."

I was amused by her comment because it reflects two frequently held misconceptions about soy. I call the first misconception the "all or nothing principle." Some people think that if they use soy, they must stop drinking cow's milk and opt for a vegetarian or vegan lifestyle. In reality, it is not a mutually exclusive relationship. Soy products can be assimilated into your regular diet.

The second misconception is that the only way to enjoy the benefits of soy is to convert to drinking only soy milk or eating tofu. In fact, today there is a vast array of soy products on the market from which to choose. From soy cereals to yogurt to burgers, there is literally something for everyone. After all, where there's a will, there's a way.

When my clients try soy, they generally fall into one of two distinct groups, those who immediately like and embrace soy and

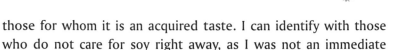

those for whom it is an acquired taste. I can identify with those who do not care for soy right away, as I was not an immediate convert to soy myself.

When I decided I wanted to try soy, I made the same mistake many soy novices make. I went out, purchased the first brand of soy milk I could find, brought it home, poured it into a glass, and drank it. Ugh! I hated it. I did not care for the taste, sight, or smell of it, but what was I going to do with the carton I'd just bought? I decided to cook and bake with the soy milk until it was gone, and I soon discovered that it was pretty good this way. Initially, that is all I did to get soy into my diet, and if that's as far as you get, that's okay.

After a few months of cooking and baking with soy milk, I decided I wanted to do more, so I experimented with different brands and found one I liked even better. Then I became really brave and poured it over my cereal—not straight, at first. I started out mixing it half and half with skim milk, and over the course of 6 months, I gradually increased the proportion of soy milk until I arrived at full strength.

Do I drink soy milk straight out of the glass? No, I still do not like it that way. However, I have incorporated other soy products into my diet. Some of my favorites include soy flour (replace ¼ of the flour in recipes), soy nuts on my salad, tofu (in stir-fry and eggless-salad sandwiches), soy-cheese slices, and soy burgers. Do I still drink skim milk? Yes I do, and I love it.

Whether you make the commitment to try soy because of its antioxidant properties or its phytohormonal effects, the health benefits abound. A review of the literature reveals quite a bit on the merits of soy, with the bulk of the research focusing on soy's role in menopause, osteoporosis, heart disease, and breast cancer. Let's briefly examine each issue.

The reason soy works to stabilize and normalize hormonal fluctuations is because it is a phytoestrogen (plant estrogen). One biologically active class of compounds in soy is called isoflavones (genistein, daidzein, and equol). The isoflavones function in our bodies like the weakest form of estrogen, estriol. They can mimic the effects of estriol because their structure is chemically similar enough to estriol to allow them to bind with the estrogen-receptor sites on the cells throughout the body. This can quell menopausal changes, particularly hot flashes and night sweats.

Another advantage of the ability of the isoflavones to bind to the receptor sites is that it is believed that they displace more potent estrogens so that the body uses the weaker ones first and excretes the excess stronger estrogens.

Initially, much of the interest surrounding soy and menopause came from observing the differences between women in Japan and those in Western societies. Japanese women report much less of a problem with hot flashes and seem to transition through menopause more easily. Researchers have concluded that much of this can be attributed to the Japanese diet, which is high in fiber and low in fat, and includes some form of soy at every meal.

One study conducted using 58 postmenopausal women experiencing at least 14 hot flashes per week reported a 40 percent reduction in hot flashes by including 45 grams of soy flour daily.[3] Another Italian study concluded that using soy-protein supplements daily significantly reduced the frequency and severity of hot flashes after 6 weeks.[4]

In conjunction with calcium, soy seems to play a pivotal role in bone mineralization. Soy's bone-preserving effects may stem from a two-pronged approach. First of all, soy's plant protein may trigger less calcium excretion than does animal protein. Second, the isoflavones may nurture bone tissue in the same way estrogen does.

In fact, a small 1996 study conducted at the University of Illinois at Urbana-Champaign revealed that the postmenopausal women not on HRT who received the most isoflavones (90 mg per day) enjoyed a slight increase in bone density after 6 months, as compared to the other study groups.[5] This could explain why Asian women whose diets are higher in isoflavone content but low in calcium are less likely to develop osteoporosis than their Western counterparts. These are preliminary studies that I'm sure will stimulate more research scrutinizing the relationship between isoflavones and osteoporosis.

Table 7.4: Approximate Isoflavone Content of Selected Foods

Soy food	Total Isoflavones (mg)
Soy milk (½ cup)	10
Tofu (½ cup)	38
Tempeh (½ cup)	60
Miso (½ cup)	40
Textured soy protein (dry, ½ cup)	56
Soy flour (½ cup)	88
Mature soy beans (uncooked, ½ cup)	175.6
Roasted soy beans (½ cup)	167

Source: 1999 Soy Foods Directory

Yes, isoflavones are cardioprotective. They lower total cholesterol, LDL, and triglycerides. In 1995, a meta-analysis of 38 studies showed that participants who consumed an average of 47 grams of soy protein daily lowered their total cholesterol by 9 percent and their LDL cholesterol by 13 percent.[6] In fact, the FDA now allows manufacturers of soy food products to display on their labels the heart-healthy benefits of eating 25 grams of soy protein daily. Keep in mind, though, that using soy must be part of a low-fat, high-fiber diet in order to lower lipid levels.

Right about now you're probably wondering, "If soy products contain all of the benefits of estrogen, do they also contain all of the risks?" The answer, at this time, is that they do not appear to carry the same risks as estrogen. However, in order to definitively make this claim, we need the benefit of a few more well-controlled studies.

Even though phytoestrogens mimic the effects of estriol, it is believed that they do not stimulate uterine tissue or increase the risk of uterine cancer. In fact, soy products seem to lower overall cancer risk.

Until recently, soy was not believed to have a proliferative effect on breast cells either. However, a handful of studies have made this association unclear. A few studies have demonstrated an increase in the number of breast cells while using soy supplements. It is not known if this affects breast cancer risk. It is interesting to note that postmenopausal Japanese women with breast cancer have a better prognosis than do postmenopausal American women, regardless of the tumor stage at diagnosis. Researchers speculate that the phytoestrogens arrest the growth of breast cancer cells.

Researchers also have found that vegetarians and women living in areas of low breast cancer incidence have higher urinary lignan levels than do women living in areas of high breast cancer incidence.[7] (Lignans are another class of phytoestrogens found mainly in flax, whole grains, and some fruits and vegetables.) However, because more research is needed in this area, some experts caution breast cancer survivors against consuming too much soy. Unfortunately, "too much" has yet to be defined. Again, there have been studies that do not bear out these concerns regarding "too much," so some experts do not exercise this caution.

If breast cancer survivors wish to use soy, I suggest they consume soy products rather than take soy supplements. It is easier to ingest high doses of isoflavones via pills rather than via food. Also, there could be dozens of active compounds in soy products that have yet to be identified, and if they haven't been isolated, they will not be found in the supplements. If you are a breast cancer survivor and are taking Tamoxifen, be aware that it is not known how soy may or may not affect this medication.

It is true that the benefits of soy abound, but how does this knowledge affect women on a daily basis? For example, how much soy should we eat? Here the information is not very clear, because not only do researchers use different amounts of soy in their studies, but the amounts they use differ based on which disorder the researchers are studying, be it osteoporosis, heart disease, or another.

Most sources recommend 30–50 mg of isoflavones a day for menopausal women. This may be based on the amount consumed by the average Asian woman. Andrew Weil, M.D., recommends con-

---

Table 7.5: Soy Smoothie

(265 calories, 15 grams of protein, 3 grams of fat,
44.5 grams of carbohydrate)

1 cup soy milk

½–1 cup berries — strawberries, blackberries, raspberries, cranberries, etc. (3 tbsp. of juice concentrate, such as cranberry, raspberry, orange, etc., can be substituted)

2 tbsp. soy protein drink mix

1 tbsp. honey to taste (or sugar substitute)

1 tsp. vanilla

4–6 ice cubes

Place all ingredients in blender and blend until ice is crushed. The extra can be frozen.

---

suming one serving of soy a day to reduce breast cancer risk, one to two servings a day to alleviate menopausal changes, two to four servings a day to lower cholesterol levels, and four or more servings a day to decrease osteoporosis risk.[8] In any event, be sure to introduce soy products into your diet gradually, as they can cause gas.

Table 7.4 will help you calculate the isoflavone content of various soy products. Sometimes this information is listed on the label, or you can contact the manufacturer to request the information.

I also have included the recipe for my favorite soy drink. I am constantly modifying it to suit my tastes and needs, but the basic recipe is pretty simple. (See Table 7.5 above.) For more information on using soy products, including almost 100 easy-to-prepare recipes, read *The Natural Estrogen Diet* by Dr. Lana Liew with Linda Ojeda, Ph.D.

Another food that imparts similar benefits to soy is flaxseed. These tiny golden or brown seeds are a great source of fiber, lignans, and omega-3 fatty acids. Flaxseed can alleviate some menopausal changes, improve cholesterol levels, provide the brain with essential fatty acids, and regulate bowel functioning.

Flaxseed must be ground in order for you to receive the health benefits. If the seeds are eaten whole, they will pass through the body undigested. Keep them refrigerated and grind only a small amount at a time so they don't become rancid. An electric coffee bean grinder works very well. Ground flaxseed has a slightly nutty flavor and can be sprinkled on peanut butter toast and hot or cold cereals; added to pancake, muffin, and sweet bread batter; or mixed into a soy smoothie drink.

Fat Is Not a Dirty Word

Despite what most people believe, fat is not a nutritional villain. It's not as if we can eliminate fat and suddenly become healthier. In fact, quite the opposite is true. Fat performs certain vital functions in our bodies. It is necessary for energy production, regulation of body temperature, hormone synthesis, and vitamin storage. However, too much fat in the diet has been linked to cancer—particularly colon, breast, ovarian, uterine, and prostate cancers—and to heart disease.

I believe that most Americans want to lower their fat intake and are aware of some of the dietary guidelines regarding total fat, saturated fat, and cholesterol. Translating this desire into practice—what we eat for breakfast, lunch, and supper—is another matter.

For example, you may know that you are supposed to consume less than 30 percent of your calories from fat, but what does this mean when eating supper? When you cook your meals or look down at your plate, can you tell what percentage of your calories are from fat? Most people cannot. With that in mind, the following suggestions should help you understand the basics of fat and how to implement a low-fat diet.

Step 1—Eat a diet low in total fat. Your total fat intake should not exceed 30 percent of your total daily calories. As a general rule, the average woman who consumes 2,000 calories a day can

Table 7.6: Calorie Requirement Chart

	Sedentary	Moderate	Active
Overweight	20–25 cal/kg	30 cal/kg	35 cal/kg
Normal	30 cal/kg	35 cal/kg	40 cal/kg
Underweight	30 cal/kg	40 cal/kg	45–50 cal/kg

Example:

1. Target weight = (150 pounds)/2.2 = 68 kilograms (kg)
2. 68 kg x 25 cal/kg (overweight, sedentary activity level)
   = 1,700 calories per day
3. 1,700 calories x 0.20 (.20%) = 340 calories from fat
4. (340 calories from fat)/9 = 38 grams

---

eat 44 grams a fat daily and maintain a low-fat (below 20 percent) diet. The exact number of fat grams varies according to activity level and weight. A dietitian can help you determine your needs, or you can use the chart below to help you. In either case, it is much simpler when reading labels to have a target number of fat grams rather than trying to calculate percentages.

Find Your Daily Calorie and Fat-Gram Budget

1. Select a realistic target weight. Convert that weight from pounds to kilograms by dividing the number of pounds by 2.2.

2. Refer to the Calorie Requirement Chart in Table 7.6. (1) From the far-left column, choose whether you are currently overweight, normal, or underweight. (2) Next, gauge your activity level. Moderate activity would entail exercising for 15 to 60 minutes three to five times per week at 50 percent to 80 percent of your estimated maximum heart rate; sedentary and active levels can be assessed accordingly. (3) From these two factors, find where you fall on the chart. This number equals how many calories per kilogram of body weight you

require daily. (4) Finally, estimate your total daily caloric requirement by multiplying the number form the chart times your target weight in kilograms. You have now estimated your daily calorie needs.

3. Multiply your daily caloric need by 20 percent to 30 percent to determine how many calories per day should come from fat. Most nutritional authorities recommend limiting your fat intake to no more than 30 percent of your total daily calorie intake. Twenty percent often is recommended for weight loss.

4. Divide the total fat calories per day by 9 to get the number of fat grams per day. (One gram of fat provides 9 calories.) You have now estimated your daily fat allowance.

Step 2—Reduce saturated fat. Equally important as the amount of fat you eat is the type of fat you eat. Saturated fat sends your cholesterol and triglyceride levels soaring and may cause cellular damage. Most saturated fat is derived primarily from animal sources, such as beef, pork, lamb, poultry, whole milk, butter, cream, ice cream, and cheese. The remainder comes from certain plant oils, such as coconut and palm oils, as well as chocolate. Therefore, be sure to choose lean meats, eat more poultry and seafood, and use low-fat or nonfat dairy products. Saturated fat should comprise no more than 10 percent of your daily calorie intake. In other words, the average American woman eating 2,000 calories a day should get no more than 22 grams of fat from saturated sources.

Since you should be reducing saturated fat in your diet, you can substitute unsaturated fats, such as monounsaturated and polyunsaturated oils, for saturated fat. Olive, canola, and peanut oils all are monounsaturated fats. When factored into your total daily fat allotment, they seem to lower LDL cholesterol. Some people mistakenly believe that they can eat unlimited amounts of these oils because they're "good for you," but excess fat is excess fat, no matter which type of fat it is.

The other vegetable oils—such as corn, sesame, safflower, sunflower, and soy—are polyunsaturated in nature.

As if it isn't difficult enough to keep these terms straight, one more term has been thrown into the equation—trans fatty acids. In order to grasp this concept, it is necessary to understand the chemical definition of the terms saturated and unsaturated.

Hydrogenation is a process that converts unsaturated fats into saturated fats. It does this by flooding the unsaturated fat with hydrogen atoms. The purpose of this chemical reaction is to change fats that are liquid at room temperature (for example, vegetable oil) to fats that are solids at room temperature (for example, shortening). The byproducts of this process are trans fatty acids. Research indicates that they can raise LDL cholesterol in the same manner as do saturated fats and may dramatically raise the risk of coronary artery disease. Trans fatty acids can be found in shortenings and stick margarine. As a general rule, tub and liquid margarines have fewer trans fatty acids.

Step 3—Limit high-cholesterol foods. Although total fat intake and saturated fat intake bear the greatest impact on cholesterol level, dietary cholesterol also is a contributing factor. Since your body is capable of manufacturing all the cholesterol it needs, exogenous cholesterol (that obtained through diet) should not exceed 300 mg per day.

Cholesterol comes only from foods of animal origin, such as beef, pork, lamb, poultry, fish, dairy products, and eggs. The recommendations for eating eggs have flip-flopped over the years, but they now stand at limiting eggs to four per week. Keep in mind that the yolk is what contains the cholesterol, so if you remove it you also remove the cholesterol content.

Step 4—Include omega fatty acids in your diet. More information is becoming available on the health benefits of omega fatty acids. Studies suggest that they may help lower the risk of heart disease and maintain cognitive integrity. Rich sources of omega-3 and omega-6 fatty acids include seafood (salmon, mackerel, tuna), walnuts, and flaxseed. (Flax meal is lower in fat.) These fatty acids are valuable contributions to total fat intake.

Step 5—Read food labels. Become aware of what you are buying and eating. This begins with label reading. Many label readers focus solely on calories, which are only one piece of the puzzle. Scrutinize total fat; saturated fat; and trans-, mono-, and polyunsaturated fats, if listed. This same principle applies to analyzing recipes, which is becoming easier since many now contain a nutritional breakdown. Once you become familiar with fat sources, it also will become easier to make healthier selections when eating out at restaurants.

The "Weigh" We Were

What woman in America has not been on at least one diet in her lifetime? The struggle of balancing a realistic body image against an idealized notion of how women should look is a full-time job for most women. Some women freely admit that their life is one perpetual fad diet after another.

Why are they unsuccessful at achieving permanent weight loss? I truly believe that the reasons people overeat and underexercise are as individual and complex as the people themselves. Most people acknowledge that they know what they "should" do, but putting it into practice is another issue altogether.

Tapping into what motivates each person is essential to modifying lifestyle habits. Working with trained professionals—for example, a psychologist or registered dietitian—is extremely beneficial to "diet lifers." There also are many books on the market that can educate as well as support your new lifestyle goals. A few of my favorites are *Outsmarting the Female Fat Cell* and *Outsmarting the Midlife Fat Cell,* both by Debra Waterhouse, R.D., and *Make the Connection,* by Oprah Winfrey and Bob Greene.

I also believe that common sense goes a long way, so I have outlined a few suggestions for losing and maintaining weight. These are followed by a formula used to calculate body mass index (BMI), which has replaced the height/weight tables previously used.

- Be choosier about what you eat. Eat more fruits, vegetables, and whole grains. When choosing dairy products, be sure to buy reduced-fat or nonfat products. When selecting meats, strive for leaner cuts, and reduce overall consumption of red meat.

- Pay attention to your portions. Sometimes, our eyes are bigger than our stomachs. Also, become familiar with typical serving sizes. For example, one serving of meat is only the size of a deck of cards—before cooking.

- Become friends with fiber. Read labels and gradually increase your fiber intake to 25 to 35 grams per day. Good sources of fiber include legumes, dried fruits, fresh fruits and vegetables, whole grains, breads, and cereals.

- Tune in to your body's cues. Eat when you are actually hungry as opposed to when you are feeling some emotion, and stop eating when you begin to feel full—not stuffed. Keep in mind that it takes 20 minutes for satiety to register in the brain, so eat slowly and watch your portions.

Table 7.7: Body Mass Index (BMI)

The Body Mass Index (BMI) is a measurement of weight as it compares to height. It is the measurement that most nutritionists now use, instead of height/weight tables. While BMI charts do exist, the index also can be calculated mathematically.

- Divide your weight in pounds by your height in inches.
- Take that number and divide it again by your height in inches.
- Multiply that number by 703.
- Locate your results below.

      Less than 18.5—underweight

      18.5–24.9—normal weight

      25–29.9—overweight

      30–39.9—obese

      40+—extremely obese

▣ Identify your eating triggers. Food often fills a void or satisfies an emotional need. Preventing overeating (or undereating) due to feeling lonely, sad, angry, or happy begins with recognizing this association.

▣ Dine "in" more than "out." Eating out frequently is the kiss of death for people trying to eat a low-fat, high-fiber diet. Even if you choose the healthiest entrée, it may still be higher in fat and calories than is desirable. Since restaurant portions tend to be large, a helpful rule of thumb is to divide the food in half and either take the rest home for another meal or split it with someone. You also may wish to request a lunch-size portion, which generally is smaller.

Super Supplements

For years, the question of whether or not to take vitamins has caused much controversy. Yet it still remains basically unanswered. However, the scales are finally beginning to tip in favor of taking vitamins. More research is demonstrating the usefulness of taking supplements. I personally endorse the responsible use of supplements in addition to a healthy diet. Remember, they are called supplements, not replacements. Do not use supplements as a means of justifying a nutrient-poor diet.

When discussing supplements with my clients, I assess their health and lifestyles, and together we determine their individual needs. In some cases, it is simply a matter of recommending antioxidants; in other cases, a more in-depth approach to fortifying the person's immune system or managing specific symptoms is required.

The one constant I stress in all of my interactions with clients is responsibility. That means the client needs to become knowledgeable about the supplements they plan to use. Such knowledge includes dosages, interactions, and side effects.

If healthy adult women are interested in using antioxidants, I suggest the following basic daily guidelines:

Mixed carotenoids—15,000–25,000 IU

Vitamin C—500–1,000 mg (doses divided throughout the day)

Vitamin E—(d-alpha tocopherol or mixed d tocopherols) 400–800 IU

Selenium—200–400 mcg

4. Are You Having Fun Yet?

If you are asking yourself "who has time for fun?" then you are probably the person who needs it the most. I don't know about you, but I cannot get through a day without at least one person telling me how "stressed out" they are. (And to be perfectly honest, sometimes the person is myself.)

We truly have become a society suffering from stress-related problems—headaches, digestive disturbances, difficulty swallowing, neckaches and backaches, anxiety, insomnia, stress-related overeating, fatigue, emotional problems—and it is believed that stress is a contributing factor to serious and chronic illness. Worse yet are those people who do not recognize the distress signals their bodies are sending out.

SUSAN is a 27-year-old attorney I met at a party. Upon discovering that I was a nurse, she began telling me her health history. She stated that she was plagued by frequent headaches, endured almost daily digestive trouble, suffered extreme fatigue, and periodically experienced a "flutter" in her chest.

After performing a battery of tests, Susan's physician gave her a "clean bill of health," as well as some medicine for symptomatic relief. I'm sure what he actually meant was that he could not find a pathological reason for her symptoms, but personally I would not have gone so far as to give her a clean bill of health. In fact, she looked me straight in the eyes and said, "I still feel awful."

I then asked her to give me a snapshot of her life. I wanted to know what a typical day was like for her. To summarize, she told me she worked 60 hours a week and brought work home on the weekends. Due to her schedule and the nature of her work, she dined out on a daily basis with clients and colleagues. When she was at home, she generally grabbed something quick to eat. This translated into a high-fat diet. In fact, talking with her revealed that her idea of a balanced meal was polishing off a pint of Ben & Jerry's ice cream after a TV dinner. At least she was honest about her eating habits. The only exercise she reported was walking to and from the elevator at work, and she got only 6 hours of sleep every night.

When I asked her what she did for fun, she listed a number of work-related activities designed to entertain clients. For myself, I don't care how enjoyable the activity is; if I'm doing it on behalf of my employer, then it is work.

After assessing her lifestyle, it became painfully obvious that Susan's body could no longer withstand the neglect. It could compensate for only so long before screaming out the message, "Help me!"

Susan needed to make some changes, so we scheduled an appointment for her to come to my office, and together we devised her "life plan." The plan included learning a new way of eating, incorporating exercise into her daily routine, and learning how to establish some boundaries so she did not bite off more work than she could handle. It also included building a social network. Identifying activities that she enjoyed and people she liked being around was an integral part of her life plan.

Although she seemed highly motivated, once she left my office I had no way of knowing if she would actually implement her life plan. Three months later, she stopped in to see me and I almost did not recognize her. She looked like a new person and she said she'd never felt better.

Susan told me that of all the changes she'd made, making herself a priority and taking time for herself was the most important. Giving herself permission to relax and have fun made all the difference in the world. She had made an investment in herself, and she was now enjoying the payoff.

Like Susan, many of us have lost balance in our lives. If you are not making enough time for rest and relaxation, you will not be in a state of harmony. Pretty soon, your mind and body will rebel, and that rebellion will be reflected in your health.

Imagine life as a balance scale—the kind you may have used in science class to measure substances. On one side of the scale you have energy zappers, and on the other side you have energy enhancers. In order to achieve balance, the two sides must even out.

What are your energy zappers? They could be related to work—such as feeling overwhelmed or dissatisfied with your job, believing that your coworkers are not pulling their fair share of the workload, or thinking your boss is an idiot.

What about your situation at home? Are you involved in at least a few loving, supportive relationships? Are you putting in the "second shift"—cooking, cleaning, laundry, helping the kids with their homework, driving the family "taxi," or caring for aging parents?

And then there are those miscellaneous frustrations, such as the crazy driver exhibiting road rage who cuts you off and nearly causes an accident, or the rude clerk at the grocery store. All of these things drain your energy, so it is important to restore your energy as well.

What, then, are your energy enhancers? Do you even have any? Ask yourself these questions: When was the last time I had fun? What do I do to enjoy myself? How do I relax?

Activities such as dancing, playing cards, going to movies, playing golf, listening to music, reading a book, and getting together with friends are just a few examples of ways to relax. Make relaxation a priority, so that you do it regularly. Keep in mind that relaxation isn't frivolous. After all, relaxing is vital to maintaining your mental and physical well-being.

5. No Stinkin' Thinkin'

We all know them don't we? Those Gloomy Guses of the world who seem to walk around with perpetual frowns on their faces and black clouds hanging over their heads. These people just exude negativity, and what's worse is that it can be contagious.

When you see one of them walking toward you, what do you do? You think, "Oh no, here comes doom and gloom." You inwardly groan, your shoulders sag, and your whole demeanor changes. If you must interact with these people on a regular basis, they can suck the very life force out of you—if you let them. These are the people the world refers to as pessimists. Their negative attitudes and beliefs cause them to focus on everything that is wrong rather than on everything that is right.

Here is a cute story that illustrates the difference between an optimist and a pessimist. There were two little boys; one was an optimist and the other was a pessimist. They put the pessimist in a room full of toys and the optimist in a room full of horse manure. One hour later, they checked on the two boys. They noticed that the pessimist was crying and asked him, "What's wrong?" He said, "One of my toys is broken." Then they looked in on the optimist, who was smiling and shoveling away. They asked him what he was doing and he replied, "Well, with all of this manure, I figured there must be a pony in here somewhere!"

What a difference perception makes. Cultivating a positive attitude and a sense of humor are essential to our health and happiness. Think about a person who is cheerful, upbeat, and pleasant. Upon first meeting this person, you might be inclined to think, "Boy, I wish I had her life. She's so carefree. She must not have a problem in the world."

Ironically, that is rarely the case. In fact, oftentimes positive people have confronted many obstacles in their lives. They have overcome adversity and as a result have developed their inner strength and wisdom, and they have managed to maintain a great outlook on life. These people are optimists.

Not only do optimists have better-functioning immune systems, but they are a joy to be around. We should try to surround ourselves with as many of these people as possible, especially since their good moods can be infectious.

Research shows that smiling—a big grin, not a perfunctory smile—actually boosts your mood. The simple act of smiling flexes the big muscles in your face, which triggers the same brain activity that occurs when you're feeling naturally happy. So even if you do not start your day in a good mood, by smiling you can cajole yourself into one.

The bottom line is that you can be a more relaxed, positive, pleasant person. We all have that potential. And doing so is a win-win situation. People will like being around you, and you will like being around you as well. I truly believe that what you put out comes back to you tenfold. So wouldn't you rather put out positive energy?

6. Roses Are Red...

Maintaining loving, nurturing relationships is vital to your health and well-being. A great deal of research indicates that people who feel deeply connected to others, especially to a mate, enjoy a lower incidence of disease, higher survival rates, and increased longevity. Here is yet another reason to treasure our families and friends.

Oftentimes, however, we take our friends and family members for granted. For example, when you've had a bad day, who feels the effects? Your husband? Your children? Poor Fido? It's ironic. These are the very ones who love us the most, yet they also are the ones we tend to treat the worst.

I don't believe this behavior is necessarily intentional. Instead, I think it is more a reflection of the stress and unhappiness in our lives. Still, there is no excuse for treating others badly, not even strangers. It's possible to forge fleeting connections with them, too.

That's what random acts of kindness are all about—doing something for someone you don't even know, just for the sake of helping them and not because you expect something in return. You do it for the sheer altruism of the act.

A random act of kindness doesn't have to be something profound or time-consuming. Holding open a door, helping someone pick up something they've dropped, allowing a car in the other lane to merge ahead of you, and rescuing an animal are simple examples that can make a big difference in someone's day—and hopefully trigger the ripple effect.

7. Sorry Seems to Be the Hardest Word

Forgiveness is the fragrance the violet sheds
on the heel that has crushed it. — Mark Twain

Doesn't that quote capture the essence of forgiveness? Forgiveness means acknowledging that someone has wronged you, and then eventually finding it in your heart to forgive that person anyway. This is an alien concept to someone who won't even consider forgiving.

It is easy to say you can forgive, but following through on it is a different story. Why are people so resistant to forgiveness? There are probably several reasons, but two immediately come to mind.

The first reason is that it is easier to harbor a grudge and feel justified about it than it is to exert the emotional energy required to work out your differences with another person. It can feel uncomfortable to address conflict or to extend the olive branch. Whether you are the person who needs to accept the responsibility and say, "I'm sorry. I really screwed up this time" or the person who decides to be big enough to say, "I don't want to sacrifice our relationship over this dispute. Let's try to work it out," there is an element of risk involved. I call this the vulnerability factor. Often, when making amends, there is a fear of rejection or of being hurt again.

The second reason that inhibits people from gravitating toward reconciliation is that we equate forgiving someone with condoning the person's actions. Forgiving doesn't imply condoning. Forgiveness means recognizing the pain and, despite everything else, working through it and releasing it. In doing so, you are denying its destructive power over your life. It does not mean that you agree with the person's actions.

When the dust settles, forgiveness doesn't even mean that the person has to be a part of your life. It simply means relinquishing the control held over your life by anger and hurt, so that you can be at peace. Remember, forgiveness is not about the other person or even about the situation that triggered the anger and hurt. It is about your own ability to heal and move forward, to grow and transcend so that anger and other intense emotions don't negatively affect the quality of your life on a daily basis.

8. Don't Become a Pressure Cooker

Do you often find yourself feeling overwhelmed, rushed, and short-tempered? Do you feel like your life is one big "to do" list? Are you the one complaining that there aren't enough hours in a day? If the answers are yes, stop and ask yourself these simple questions: Why am I in this predicament, and what can I do to change it?

Normally, when I pose these questions to people, they become defensive and begin to say things like, "Well I gotta..." and "I have to..." and "I should...." While I understand that everyone has responsibilities, I also understand that we all have choices. The will to choose how we respond to situations, how we perceive our lives, and how we spend our time is within our control.

The quality of your day should not be defined by the quantity of tasks you accomplish. There will always be more work to be done. It will never all get done, so instead of feeling like a horse at the starting gate from the moment the alarm goes off in the morning, why not take the time to enjoy the people you are with and devote all your attention to what you are doing at the present moment? Soon, you will be able to focus not only on what you did accomplish—instead of on what you didn't get done—but more importantly, on the beauty and joy that each new day holds. Not surprisingly, you will become a more relaxed person and may even rediscover your sense of humor.

Remember the adage "Life is too short to be taken seriously"? I believe that statement is very true. It has been noted that the average child laughs 300 times a day, but the average adult laughs only four to eight times a day. What happens to us during adulthood? How do we lose that natural exuberance of childhood? Is it because we begin thinking that our lives are full of too many important and serious matters? What better reason to experience joy!

Unfortunately, many of us don't learn this lesson until we are confronted by significant adversity or until we reach midlife and begin the introspection process. Whatever the impetus, it is very liberating to realize that it's not necessary to be perfect, we all have limitations, it's okay to say no, and there is always enough time.

9. Transcend and Transform: Explore Your Spirituality

We are not human beings having a spiritual experience;
we are spiritual beings having a human experience.
— Pierre Teilhard de Chardin

At some point in time, whether due to a crisis or the aging process, we all begin scrutinizing our lives. We may ask ourselves such questions as "Is this all there is to life? What's my purpose? Have I made a difference?" I believe that discovering answers to questions like these ultimately deepens and advances our spiritual development.

Many of us suppress or even deny our spirituality, as if it were not the very essence of our being. Some people shy away from spiritual exploration, citing "religious reasons." They state that they do not want to become religious fanatics or that exploration is against their religious beliefs.

Regardless of religious affiliation, I believe that spirituality is about who you are and how you live your life. It is about recognizing your life force and letting that force guide you.

Think about it. Do you live what you believe? Do you pray or go to a place of worship vowing to do God's work, only to go home and forget to exercise forgiveness with your partner? Or do you go to work and forget to exercise tolerance with your coworkers?

These situations are life lessons we learn if we are attuned to them when they present themselves. We all are on a spiritual journey; however, everyone's growth proceeds according to a different timetable. We can foster this development by strengthening our bond with a higher power.

How does one go about this? I pray and meditate. This increases my level of self-awareness and heightens my sensitivity to divine intervention. This helps me to walk the spiritual path on a daily basis.

While walking this path—and periodically taking a wrong turn—I have learned a great many lessons (some of them the hard way) that ultimately have enriched my life. Here are some of the truths I have encountered along the way:

- Live in the present moment.

- Exercise tolerance.

- Be a model, not a critic.

- Live well, laugh often, love much.

- Forge a connection to the divine.

- Practice forgiveness.

- Love is the basis of human existence.

- Serve others.

- Focus on the positive.

- Commune with nature.

- Let go of materialism. (It's okay to be successful, but it should not define who you are.)

All of these truths allow me to forge connections with myself, with others, and with all that is holy. Not only do they bring a sense of harmony and balance into my life, but they also pave the road to optimal health.

Research studies have demonstrated that people who feel a sense of interconnectedness with others and with a higher power are healthier and more likely to recover from serious and life-threatening illness. Indeed, there has been an explosion of scientific information linking prayer to health—both our own health and the health of others. Studies prove that prayer for oneself—petitionary prayer—and prayer on behalf of others—intercessory prayer—promote health, enhance recovery, and increase survival.

10. Be a Proactive Patient

Do you watch television? If so, think back to one of the numerous police shows that you may have seen. What is the first thing the police officer says to a criminal being arrested? The officer reads the criminal his rights: "You have the right to remain silent. Anything you do say can and will be used against you in a court of law...."

Now imagine the same thing happening in your doctor's office. Before your doctor examines you, she would read you your rights. What might she say to you? I envision it going something like this: "You have the right not to remain silent. Everything you say can and will be considered important. You have the right to a second opinion, to confidentiality, and to be treated with dignity. You have the right to a competent, caring, and communicative physician. If you find that I do not meet your needs, another doctor will be provided for you. Do you understand each of these rights as I have read them to you?"

Think about what this would accomplish. It would highlight some of your rights as a patient, help you to remain in control, and empower you to recognize that what you have to say is indeed important. In fact, it's crucial.

At the very foundation of being satisfied with your health care is the relationship you have with your doctor. There should be a high degree of rapport between you. I believe that the ideal situation is a 50-50 partnership with a physician who possesses the three Cs—competence, compassion, and communicativeness.

In order to achieve a situation as close to this ideal as possible, it is necessary to be aware of your patient rights and responsibilities, as well as to take the time to select a doctor carefully. Good medical care starts with going to the right doctor.

This proactive approach requires you to do some legwork when you are feeling well. Don't wait until you need a doctor to start looking for one. If you are sick or in the middle of a medical crisis, you will be less likely to make a careful, informed decision. Your goal is to find a physician that is a good match for you. Keep in mind that a doctor whom your friend considers to be a perfect match for her may not necessarily be a perfect match for you.

Finding the Right Doctor

JESSICA was a 44-year-old artist who called me because she was looking for a family doctor. When I asked her what qualities she was seeking in a physician, she was stunned into silence. Jessica replied, "I haven't given it much thought. I trust you to give me the name of a good doctor." After explaining to her that my definition of a good doctor may not be the same as hers, and that I couldn't recommend a physician off the cuff, she agreed to give the matter more thought. The two of us explored her needs and the characteristics that she wanted in a doctor. We were then able to devise a list of potential candidates.

Selecting a doctor does not require a medical degree. It does, however, require careful consideration. The following five-step plan will provide you with some guidance when looking for a doctor.

Step 1—Decide what kind of doctor you need. Before the onset of managed care, the question to ask yourself was, "Do I need a family doctor or a specialist for this problem?" Today, this decision is not always in your hands. Regardless of insurance status, I have always endorsed having a primary-care physician. This does not mean you can't go to a specialist, if appropriate, but it just makes good sense to have someone coordinating your care, as well as someone to see for life's minor medical concerns. If you are using a specialist as your primary-care physician—for example, an OB/GYN—be sure to seek care from a certified specialist if you develop a complicated or serious problem.

Step 2—Make a list of candidates. Depending on your geographic location and the type of doctor you are looking for, this list could be pretty extensive. Gathering this information is fairly easy because most hospitals have referral services or directories of the physicians on staff. Additional sources of information include the local medical society, library (look for directories of physicians and medical specialists), phone book, and university medical schools. If you are relocating, don't forget to ask your current doctor for advice. It also is a good idea to ask your friends, relatives, and people who work in health care for a referral, but don't just ask for the doctor's name. Find out specifically what the person likes or dislikes about the doctor. Don't simply accept the answer at face value.

Step 3—Narrow the list. Streamline the list according to criteria that are important to you. Of course, this means that you will have to give some thought to exactly what you are looking for in a doctor and then prioritize those qualities. You also can categorize these criteria into "must have," "nice to have," and "optional." Then rate each doctor according to your needs. Factors that you may consider important are education, special interests, hospital privileges, partners in the practice, disciplinary action rendered against the doctor, location, hours, gender, acceptance of new patients, fees, and insurance plans accepted. The answers to many of these questions can be found by speaking to the office manager or consulting a referral service or physician directory.

Step 4—Meet the doctor. Once you have narrowed the list to a handful of candidates, it is particularly beneficial to meet the doctor. Keep in mind that you are not interviewing to be her patient; she is interviewing to be your doctor. Although this step usually requires scheduling an office visit, you may be able to gauge a physician's areas of interest, bedside manner, and philosophy by attending a class she teaches or listening to her speak at a support-group meeting, on the radio, or on television. If you do schedule an appointment with a doctor, be sure to go in prepared. You likely won't have much time, and you will want to use what time you have wisely.

Draft a list of standard questions for each doctor and record the answers. If you have a particular ailment or a chronic disease, ask the doctor about her treatment philosophy regarding that condition. Most people with chronic or serious illnesses are medically savvy about their conditions and can ask the doctor to "educate" them about a certain aspect of the disease or illness. It usually becomes obvious if the doctor has kept current on that particular problem. You also should ask about the scope of the physician's practice. How many people with your condition or similar concerns does the doctor treat?

Other areas that you may wish to address with specific questions include: her education, including continuing medical education and specialty areas; where she sends lab work and diagnostic tests for interpretation, as well as the site's reliability; how quickly you can be seen for an urgent problem, as well as the lead time needed for a routine visit; attitude regarding second opinions and complementary care; and receptivity to your being an active participant in your health care.

Step 5—Choose your doctor. After you have met with the candidates, evaluate them according to your list of criteria. How did each one score? Once you have determined their ranking, give it some more thought; only this time, use your intuition. A doctor may look good on paper, but if you have a "gut feeling" that this doctor is not the one for you, then listen to your instincts.

Remember that your goal is a caring, competent, and communicative physician, and that nothing is etched in stone. Later, if the doctor you chose does not turn out to be as she presented herself—or if you change your mind for any other reason—you don't have to stick with her. We all have made poor choices and errors in judgement, but we also have the power to correct them.

I'd like to end the section on choosing a doctor with a quote from Sir William Osler, a noted Canadian medical educator: "It is as important to know the person who has the disease as the disease the person has."

He's right. There should be more to your relationship with your doctor than simply listing your symptoms and arriving at a diagnosis. It is not unreasonable to expect your health-care provider to be competent, caring, and communicative. There are many good doctors out there—ones who embody the three Cs. You just have to take the time to find them.

Patient Rights

In your pursuit of the right doctor and the best medical care, it is crucial to be aware of your rights and responsibilities as a patient. Sometimes we lose sight of the fact that we are entitled to certain fundamental rights from our health-care providers, and that we are accountable for some specific things ourselves. For this reason, I have included two lists that serve as reminders of a few practical rights and responsibilities. I also have included questions to ask your doctor regarding medications, medical tests, and surgery that might be recommended. These should serve as guidelines in helping you make informed decisions.

You have the right to:

- Confidentiality

- Obtain another opinion

- Know the price of treatment

- Be treated with dignity

▧ Be informed

▧ Access your medical records

▧ Have a competent, caring, and communicative physician

Patient Responsibilities

You are responsible for:

▧ Taking care of yourself

▧ Being honest with your doctor (don't withhold information)

▧ Communicating assertively

▧ Reporting changes and problems in a timely manner

▧ Treating your doctor and her staff with the same courtesy you expect from them

▧ Preparing for your appointment to efficiently utilize time

▧ Complying with the treatment plan decided on by you and your doctor

▧ Having reasonable expectations

▧ Paying your bills

Questions about Medication

▧ What is the name of the medication?

▧ What is the purpose of the medication?

▧ How often should I take the medicine, and how much should I take (dosage)?

▧ Should I take it with meals or on an empty stomach?

▧ Are there any restrictions while I am on this medicine (for example, no driving)?

▧ How soon will this medicine work?

▣ Are there any special instructions about taking this medicine?

▣ Will my problem resolve without medicine?

▣ Is there an over-the-counter medicine that I can take instead of a prescription?

▣ Is there a generic substitute available?

▣ What are the potential side effects?

▣ If I experience these side effects, should I continue to take the medicine?

▣ Are there any signs or symptoms that I should report to you?

▣ What are the potential long-term effects, if any?

▣ Does this medicine interact with any other medicine or with any food?

▣ Does this medicine contain any ingredients I am allergic to?

▣ Is there any written information available about this medicine?

Questions about Medical Tests/Procedures

▣ What is the name of the test/procedure?

▣ What is the purpose of the test/procedure?

▣ What will happen during the test/procedure?

▣ Who will perform the test/procedure?

▣ How many times has this person performed this test/procedure?

▣ Where do I have to go for this test/procedure?

▣ Is the facility that will interpret the results of my test accredited by a licensing board?

⬡ What are the risks of this test/procedure?

⬡ Is there another test that can yield the same information, one that is less costly or less invasive?

⬡ What is the cost of this test/procedure, and will it be covered by my insurance plan?

⬡ Are there any special preparation procedures that need to be followed before or after the test/procedure?

⬡ Should I take my regular medicines on the day of the test/procedure?

⬡ Am I allergic to anything that will be used during the test/procedure?

⬡ Will I need someone to drive me home?

⬡ Will you contact me with the results, and if so, how soon?

⬡ If the results are abnormal, what's next?

⬡ If the results are normal, what's next?

⬡ Should I seek a second opinion before having this test/procedure?

⬡ Is there any written information available about this test/procedure?

Questions about Surgery

⬡ What is the name of the operation?

⬡ What is the purpose of the operation?

⬡ What will happen during the operation?

⬡ Who will be the primary surgeon?

⬡ Who will be the assisting surgeon?

⬡ How many times have these doctors performed this operation?

- What type of anesthesia will be used?

- Who is the anesthesiologist?

- Is this an inpatient or outpatient procedure?

- Which hospital will be used?

- How long will I be in the hospital?

- Is this surgery necessary to prevent death?

- What are the risks of this surgery?

- What are the risks of not having this surgery?

- Are there any special preparation procedures I need to follow before surgery?

- Should I take my regular medicines on the day of surgery?

- Am I allergic to anything that will be used during surgery?

- What does the recovery entail; for example, will I be limited in my activities, and how long will I be off of work?

- What is the cost of this surgery, and will my insurance pay for it?

- Should I get a second opinion?

- Is there any written information available about this surgery?

Beginning Your Journey

In this chapter I've covered the strategies you can implement to get on the road to wellness and well-being. You have the capability to create health in your life. Achieving it just requires two things. First, take a good, hard, honest look at your life, and choose to take it in a different direction. Second, remain dedicated to your cause. It might seem intimidating at first, but you don't have to take giant leaps and bounds. You can attain your goals via baby steps.

Expect that periodically you will stumble and fall back into your old habits. That's okay; it's normal. Simply pick yourself up, dust yourself off, and keep going. And always remember, falling down doesn't make you a failure; staying down does.

Chapter Highlights

- We all have the potential to create health in our lives. It begins with a commitment to ourselves. We must desire to improve our health and well-being.

- Creating health does not imply that you will never again be ill. It means placing your body in the best state to achieve optimal health and well-being.

- Examine the physical, emotional, and spiritual aspects of your life, and decide which area is a priority. Address issues relating to that particular area first. Once you feel you have successfully incorporated those changes into your life, select another area of focus. Some people may begin with nutritional concerns, while others choose to improve their attitude or engage in spiritual exploration.

- Remember that creating health is a journey, not a destination. Achieving lifelong success in this area depends upon looking at it as a way of life rather than as a short-term goal.

Doc Talk

- Consult professionals that may be instrumental in helping you attain your goals. This team of providers may include a doctor, nurse, nutritionist, psychologist, naturopathic practitioner, and clergy member.

- Discuss your medical needs with your doctor. Share your family medical history; determine a plan of health screenings; and ask questions about your current state of health, any medications you are taking, and medical procedures being recommended. Also, be sure to keep a copy of your medical records.

- Evaluate the relationship you have with your doctor/nurse practitioner. Are you satisfied with the care she provides and with her bedside manner? If not, it may be time to scout out a new clinician.

One Last Reminder

Keep in mind that even though sudden menopause may have occurred years earlier than expected, it should be viewed as another phase in your life. Like other phases in your life, it brings about change. Most likely, you will need to make adjustments in order to look and feel great, but you must realize that you *can* look and feel great. Never doubt that.

Always remember to look within yourself. Harness your inner strength and wisdom and celebrate the remarkable person that you are. Honor the divine spark that exists within you, and then go out into the world and enjoy your life as the wise and wonderful menopausal woman that you are!

Notes

Chapter 1

1. "CDC Finds Hysterectomies Increasing," *Lifelines*, journal published by the Association of Women's Health, Obstetric and Neonatal Nurses, Dec. 1999.
2. National Center for Health Statistics, Centers for Disease Control and Prevention, U.S. Department of Health and Human Services, unpublished data from the National Hospital Discharge Survey.
3. June M. Thompson, Dr. P.H., Gertrude K. McFarland, D.N.Sc., Jane E. Hirsch, M.S., and Susan Tucker, P.H.N., *Mosby's Clinical Nursing*, 3d ed. (St. Louis, MO: Mosby Publishing, 1993), p. 877.

Chapter 2

1. Patricia Kaufert, Ph.D., et al., "Women and Menopause: Beliefs, Attitudes and Behaviors," The North American Menopause Society 1997 Menopause Survey, *Menopause: The Journal of the North American Menopause Society*, vol. 5, no. 4 (1998), pp. 197–202.
2. Lila E. Nachtigall, M.D., *Estrogen* (New York: Harper Perennial, 1991), p. 60.
3. Barbara B. Sherwin, Ph.D., "Estrogen and/or Androgen Replacement Therapy and Cognitive Functioning in Surgically Menopausal Women," *Psychoneuroendocrinology*, vol. 13, no. 4 (1988), pp. 345–57.
4. Bruce S. McEwen, Ph.D., "Estrogens Regulate Brain Structure and Chemistry," speaker abstract from the North American Menopause Society Third Annual Meeting, Sept. 17–20, 1992.
5. Barbara B. Sherwin, op. cit.
6. "Hormone Replacement?" *Midlife Woman*, The Midlife Women's Network newsletter, vol. 1, no. 3, p. 2.
7. D. H. Richards, "Depression After Hysterectomy," *The Lancet*, Aug. 25, 1973, pp. 430–32.
8. D. H. Richards, "A Post-Hysterectomy Syndrome," *The Lancet*, Oct. 26, 1974, pp. 983–85.
9. "The Emotions of Midlife," *Midlife Woman*, The Midlife Women's Network newsletter, vol. 2, no. 3, p. 5.

10. Barbara B. Sherwin, op. cit.
11. Winnifred B. Cutler, Ph.D., *Hysterectomy: Before and After* (New York: Harper Perennial, 1990), pp. 255–57.

Chapter 3

1. *Building a Strong Foundation for You*, pamphlet, National Osteoporosis Foundation, Washington, D.C.
2. *Stand Up to Osteoporosis*, pamphlet, National Osteoporosis Foundation, 1994, p. 10.
3. Ibid.
4. Ibid.
5. Ibid.
6. *Osteoporosis: Can It Happen to You?*, National Osteoporosis Foundation and U.S. Administration on Aging, 1991.
7. U.S. Peventive Services Task Force, *Guide to Clinical Preventive Services*, 2d ed. (Baltimore: Williams and Wilkins, 1996), p. 510.
8. Nelson B. Watts, M.D., "Cyclical Etidronate," clinical update, reprinted from *The Osteoporosis Report*, Winter 1990.
9. *Monthly Prescribing Reference*, Abbot Laboratories, Inc., July 1999.
10. "Prevent Osteoporosis," *Health News: New England Journal of Medicine Newsletter*, vol. 4, no. 3 (Mar. 10, 1998).
11. Charles Y. C. Pak, M.D., et al., "Treatment of Postmenopausal Osteoporosis with Slow-Release Sodium Fluoride," *Annals of Internal Medicine*, vol. 123, issue 6 (Sept. 15, 1995), pp. 401–8.
12. *Stand Up to Osteoporosis*, pamphlet, National Osteoporosis Foundation, 1994, p. 11.
13. Anna De Planter Bowes and Helen Nichols Church, rev. by Jean A. Thompson, *Food Values of Portions Commonly Used*, 15th ed. (Philadelphia, PA: J.B. Lippincott Co., 1994).
14. *Getting Along with Milk*, pamphlet, National Dairy Council, 1993.
15. *NIH Consensus Statement: Optimal Calcium Intake*, vol. 12, no. 4 (June 6–8, 1994), p. 17.

Chapter 4

1. *Silent Epidemic: The Truth About Women and Heart Disease*, pamphlet, American Heart Association, 1992.
2. Leslie Laurence and Beth Weinhouse, *Outrageous Practices: The Alarming Truth About How Medicine Mistreats Women* (New York: Fawcett Columbine, 1994).
3. "Women and Heart Disease," *Wellness Letter*, University of California, Berkeley, Feb. 1992.

4. *Silent Epidemic*.
5. Marian Sandmaler, *The Healthy Heart Handbook for Women*, National Institutes of Health, 1992, p. 23.
6. Ibid.
7. "Take It to Heart," *Women's Health Connections*, vol. 3, no. 1 (April/May 1995).
8. Sandmaler, op. cit., p. 25.
9. Sandmaler, op. cit., p. 26.
10. Deborah Grady, M.D., "Trial Results Refute Cardiac Benefit of Estrogen-Progestin," *Geriatrics*, vol. 53, issue 10 (Oct. 1998), p. 15.
11. *Silent Epidemic*.
12. "Health After 50," *The Johns Hopkins Medical Letter*, vol. 8, issue 11 (Jan. 1997).

Chapter 5

1. Robert H. Garrison, Jr., M.A., R.Ph., and Elizabeth Somer, M.A., R.D., *The Nutrition Desk Reference*, 2d ed. (New Canaan, CT: Keats Publishing, 1990), pp. 101–2.
2. Garrison and Somer, op. cit., pp. 40–42.
3. "Cancer-Preventing Effect of Ginseng," *HerbalGram: The Journal of the American Botanical Council and the Herb Research Foundation*, no. 36, p. 17.
4. Arthur A. Siciliano, Ph.D., "Cranberry," *HerbalGram: The Journal of the American Botanical Council and the Herb Research Foundation*, no. 38, pp. 51–53.

Chapter 6

1. G. A. Colditz, et al., "The Use of Estrogens and Progestins and the Risk of Breast Cancer in Postmenopausal Women," *The New England Journal of Medicine*, vol. 332, no. 24 (June 15, 1995), pp. 1589–93.
2. J. L. Stanford, et al., "Combined Estrogen and Progestin Hormone Replacement Therapy in Relation to Risk of Breast Cancer in Middle-Aged Women," *Journal of the American Medical Association*, vol. 274, no. 2 (July 12, 1995), pp. 137–42.
3. "Second Opinion," *Mayo Clinic Health Letter*, Dec. 1994, p. 8.
4. John R. Lee, M.D., *What Your Doctor May Not Tell You About Menopause: The Breakthrough Book on Natural Progesterone* (New York: Warner Books, 1996), p. 271.
5. Susan Rako, M.D., "Can We Understand Testosterone as Just Another Hormone?" *Menopause News*, vol. 6, no. 2 (March/April 1996), p. 3.

6. Susan Rako, M.D., *The Hormone of Desire: The Truth About Sexuality, Menopause and Testosterone* (New York: Harmony Books, 1996).
7. C. Marwick, "Hormone Combination Treats Women's Bone Loss," *Journal of the American Medical Association*, vol. 272, no. 19 (Nov. 16, 1994), p. 1487.
8. Ibid.

Chapter 7

1. J. Michael McGinnis and William H. Foege, "Actual Causes of Death in the United States," *Journal of the American Medical Association*, vol. 270, no. 18 (Nov. 10, 1993), pp. 2207–12.
2. Bruce N. Ames, et al., "Oxidants, Antioxidants, and the Degenerative Diseases of Aging," *Procedures of the National Academy of Science USA*, vol. 90 (Sept. 1993), pp. 7915–22.
3. A. L. Murkies, et al., "Dietary Flour Supplementation Decreases Postmenopausal Hot Flushes: Effect of Soy and Wheat," *Maturitas*, vol. 21, no. 3 (April 1995), pp. 189–95.
4. G. Scambia, et al., "Clinical Effects of a Standardized Soy Extract in Postmenopausal Women: A Pilot Study," *Menopause*, vol. 7, no. 2 (Mar.–April 2000), pp. 105–11.
5. Susan Potter, et al., "Soy Protein and Isoflavones: Their Effects on Blood Lipids and Bone Density in Postmenopausal Women," *American Journal of Clinical Nutrition*, suppl., vol. 68 (1998), pp. 1375S–79S.
6. James W. Anderson, et al., "Meta-Analysis of the Effects of Soy Protein Intake on Serum Lipids," *New England Journal of Medicine*, vol. 333, no. 5 (Aug. 3, 1995), pp. 276–82.
7. D. C. Knight and J. A. Eden, "A Review of the Clinical Effect of Phytoestrogens," *Obstetrics and Gynecology*, vol. 87 (May 1996), pp. 897–904.
8. Andrew Weil, M.D., "The Joy of Soy," Self Healing newsletter, July 1997.

Appendix A: Menopause Resources

General

North American Menopause Society (NAMS)
PO Box 94527
Cleveland OH 44101-4527   (440) 442-7550
www.menopause.org

National Women's Health Network
514 Tenth St. NW, Suite 400
Washington DC 20004   (202) 347-1140
Fax: (202) 347-1168
www.womenshealthnetwork.org

Office on Women's Health, Department of Health and Human Services
200 Independence Ave. SW, Room 730B
Washington DC 20201   (202) 690-7650
Fax: (202) 205-2631
www.4woman.org

Menopausal Symptoms and Health Concerns

National Osteoporosis Foundation
1232 22nd St. NW
Washington DC 20037   (202) 223-2226
www.nof.org

American Heart Association
7272 Greenville Ave.
Dallas TX 75231   (214) 373-6300
www.americanheart.org

National Cancer Institute
www.nci.nih.gov   (800) 4-CANCER (422-6237)

Sexuality Information and Education Council of the U.S. (SIECUS)
130 West 42nd St., Suite 350
New York NY 10036   (212) 819-9770
Fax: (212) 819-9776
www.siecus.org

National Association for Continence (NASC)
PO Box 8310
Spartansburg SC 29305-8310   (800) BLADDER (252-3337)
Fax: (864) 579-7902
www.nafc.org

National Vulvodynia Association
PO Box 4491
Silver Springs MD 20914   (301) 299-0775
Fax: (301) 299-3999
www.nva.org

Simon Foundation for Continence
PO Box 835
Wilmette IL 60091   (800) 23SIMON (237-4666)
Fax: (847) 864-9758
www.simonfoundation.org

American Psychiatric Association
1400 K St. NW
Washington DC 20005   (202) 682-6000
Fax: (202) 682-6850
www.psych.org

American Psychological Association
750 First St. NE
Washington DC 20002-4242   (800) 374-2721
www.apa.org

Nutrition and Supplements

American Dietetic Association   (800) 366-1655
www.eatright.org

Flax Council
PO Box 281294
San Francisco CA 94128-1294   (800) 817-9894

Pennsylvania Soybean Board
PO Box 319
Salisbury MD 21803   (410) 742-9500
Fax: (410) 548-5824

Soyfoods Association of North America
1723 U St. NW
Washington DC 20009   (202) 387-5553

Center for Science in the Public Interest
1875 Connecticut Ave. NW, Suite 300
Washington DC 20009-5728   (202) 332-9110
Fax: (202) 265-4954
www.cspinet.org

Herb Research Foundation
1007 Pearl St., Suite 200
Boulder CO 80302   (303) 449-2265
Fax: (303) 449-7849
www.herbs.org

American Botanical Council
PO Box 144345
Austin TX 78714   (512) 926-4900
Fax: (512) 926-2345
www.herbalgram.org

Labs and Compounding Pharmacies

Aeron Life Cycles Laboratory
(performs hormonal saliva testing)
1933 Davis Street, Suite 310
San Leandro CA 94577   (800) 631-7900
www.Aeron.com

Madison Pharmacy Associates (Women's Health America)
429 Gammon Pl.
PO Box 259690
Madison WI 53725   (800) 222-4767
www.womenshealth.com

International Academy of Compounding Pharmacists
                                      (800) 927-4227

College Pharmacy   (800) 888-9358
Fax: (800) 556-5893
www.collegepharmacy.com

Patient Advocacy

American Board of Medical Specialties
1007 Church St., Suite 404
Evanston IL 60201   (800) 776-CERT (2378)
(847) 491-9091
Fax: (847) 328-3596
www.abms.org

Medical Record Privacy, Electronic Privacy Information Center
www.epic.org
Medi-Net   (888) 333-3365
www.askmedi.com
Conducts background checks that include disciplinary information on
any M.D. or D.O. in the United States

National Council for Reliable Health Information
PO Box 1276
Loma Linda CA 92354   (909) 824-4690
Fax: (909) 824-4838
www.ncahf.org

National Center for Complementary and Alternative Medicine
PO Box 8218
Silver Springs MD 20907-8218   (888) 644-6226
Fax: (301) 495-4957
www.nccam.nih.gov

People's Medical Society
462 Walnut St.
Allentown PA 18102   (800) 624-8773
Fax: (610) 770-0607
www.peoplesmed.org

Appendix B: Recommended Reading

Newsletters

Health Wisdom for Women, Christiane Northrup, M.D.,
www.drnorthrup.com

Nutrition Action, Center for Science in the Public Interest,
www.cspinet.org

Self Healing, Andrew Weil, M.D., www.drweilselfhealing.com

Wellness Letter, University of California, Berkeley, www.wellnessletter.com

Books

Anatomy of an Illness, Norman Cousins (New York: Bantam Books, 1985).

Anatomy of the Spirit, Caroline Myss (New York: Harmony Books, 1996).

Brain Longevity, Dharma Singh Khalsa, M.D., with Cameron Stauth (New York: Warner Books, 1997).

Eating Well for Optimum Health, Andrew Weil, M.D., (New York: Alfred A. Knopf, 2000).

Her Healthy Heart: A Woman's Guide to Preventing and Reversing Heart Disease Naturally, Linda Ojeda, Ph.D. (Alameda, CA: Hunter House, 1998).

The Hormone of Desire: The Truth About Sexuality, Menopause and Testosterone, Susan Rako, M.D. (New York: Harmony Books, 1996).

The HRT Solution: Optimizing Your Hormone Potential, Marla Ahlgrimm, R.P.H., and John M. Kells (Garden City Park, NY: Avery Publishing Group, 1999).

Journeys with the Cancer Conquerer: Mobilizing Mind and Spirit, Greg Anderson (Kansas City, MO: Andrews and McMeel, 1999).

Menopause Without Medicine, 4th ed., Linda Ojeda, Ph.D., (Alameda, CA: Hunter House, 2000).

The Natural Estrogen Diet: Healthy Recipes for Perimenopause and Menopause, Dr. Lana Liew with Linda Ojeda, Ph.D. (Alameda, CA: Hunter House, 1998).

Outsmarting the Midlife Fat Cell, Debra Waterhouse, M.P.H., R.D. (New York: Hyperion, 1998).

The Power of the Mind to Heal, Joan Borysenko, Ph.D., and Miroslav Borysenko, Ph.D. (Carson City, CA: Hay House, Inc., 1994).

Power Sleep, James B. Maas, Ph.D. (New York: Villard Books, 1998).

Relax: You May Only Have a Few Minutes Left, Loretta LaRoche (New York: Villard, 1998).

Screaming to Be Heard: Hormonal Connections Women Suspect...and Doctors Ignore, Elizabeth Lee Vliet, M.D. (New York: M. Evans and Company, Inc., 1995).

Spontaneous Healing, Andrew Weil, M.D., (New York: Alfred A. Knopf, 1995).

The Ten Best Tools to Boost Your Immune System, Elinor Levy, Ph.D., and Tom Monte (New York: Houghton Mifflin Company, 1997).

Women's Bodies, Women's Wisdom, Christiane Northrup, M.D. (New York: Bantam, 1998).

Index

MENOPAUSE WITHOUT MEDICINE
by Linda Ojeda, Ph.D. ... New Fourth Edition

Linda Ojeda broke new ground 15 years ago with this bestselling resource on menopause, giving women a clear understanding of menopausal changes and guidelines for effective self-care.

In this new edition she reexamines the hormone therapy debate; suggests natural remedies for depression, hot flashes, sexual changes, and skin and hair problems; and presents an illustrated basic exercise program. She also includes up-to-date information on natural sources of estrogen, including phytoestrogens, and how diet and personality affect mood swings.

352 pages ... 32 illus. ... 62 tables ... Paperback $15.95... Hardcover $25.95

THE NATURAL ESTROGEN DIET: Healthy Recipes for Perimenopause and Menopause
by Dr. Lana Liew with Linda Ojeda, Ph.D.

Two women's health and nutrition experts offer women almost 100 easy and delicious recipes that will naturally increase their estrogen levels. Each recipe includes nutritional information, such as the calorie, cholesterol, and calcium contents. The authors also provide an overview of how estrogen can be derived from the food we eat, describe which foods are the highest in estrogen content, and offer meal plan ideas.

224 pages ... 25 illus. ... Paperback ... $13.95

HER HEALTHY HEART: A Woman's Guide to Preventing and Reversing Heart Disease *Naturally*
by Linda Ojeda, Ph.D.

Almost twice as many women die from heart disease and stroke as from all forms of cancer combined. In fact, heart disease is the #1 killer of American women ages 44 to 65, yet until now most of the research and attention has been given to men. This book fills this gap by addressing the unique aspects of heart disease in women and the natural ways to combat it. Dr. Ojeda explains how women can prevent heart disease, whether they take hormone replacement therapy (HRT) or not. She provides detailed information on how to reduce the risk of heart disease through diet, physical activity, and stress management.

352 pages .... Paperback $14.95 .... Hardcover $24.95

WOMEN'S SEXUAL PASSAGES: Finding Pleasure and Intimacy at Every Stage of Life *by* Elizabeth Davis

In this completely revised edition of her earlier book *Women, Sex, and Desire,* Davis unravels the mystery of how and why women's desire changes in the course of a lifetime under the influence of biological rhythms, hormones, and menstruation; pregnancy, birth, and child rearing; cultural attitudes, menopause, and aging.

Davis focuses on ways for women to truly understand their sexuality. She looks at the effects of stress, overwork, major life events, relationship upheaval, and sexual abuse. New chapters address sexual awakening and sex in the later years, and how hormonal changes at menopause are linked to increased insight and assertiveness.

288 pages ... 8 illus. ... Paperback $15.95

SEXUAL PLEASURE: Reaching New Heights of Sexual Arousal and Intimacy *by* Barbara Keesling, Ph.D.

This bestselling book is for all people who are interested in enhancing their sex lives. Written in a warm, encouraging tone, it helps readers to recognize the key to fulfilling sex: becoming aware of their own sensuality and learning to focus on their own arousal before trying to please their partner.

The exercises in *Sexual Pleasure* take readers from simple body-image and self-caress techniques to intense levels of arousal, orgasm, and prolonged release. The open approach of the book is conveyed artistically in sensual photographs that complement the text.

224 pages ... 14 illus. ... Paperback ... $12.95 ... Hardcover $21.95

MAKING LOVE BETTER THAN EVER: Reaching New Heights of Passion and Pleasure After 40
by Barbara Keesling, Ph.D.

Great sex is not reserved for people under 40. With maturity comes the potential for a multi-faceted loving that draws from all we are. In this book, Barbara Keesling shows how loving touch has the power to heighten sexual response and expand sexual potential; reduce anxiety and increase health and well-being; build self-esteem and improve body image; open the lines of communication; and promote playfulness, spontaneity, and a natural sense of joy.

208 pages ... 14 b/w photos ... Paperback $13.95 ... Hardcover $24.95

All prices subject to change

THE COMPLETE GUIDE TO JOSEPH H. PILATES' TECHNIQUES OF PHYSICAL CONDITIONING: Applying the Principles of Body Control

by Allan Menezes, Founder of the Pilates Institute of Australasia

This comprehensive book includes a complete floor program (no special equipment needed) that guides readers through basic, intermediate, and advanced routines, with detailed descriptions of each exercise and step-by-step photographs. There is a special section on relieving back, ankle, and shoulder pain, and insights on how the work can be adapted by athletes. Worksheets are provided to record progress, and an introduction gives the history and legacy of Joseph Pilates.

208 pages ... 191 b/w photos ... 80 illus. & charts ... Paperback $19.95 ... Spiral Bound $26.95

GET FIT WHILE YOU SIT: Easy Workouts from Your Chair

by Charlene Torkelson

Here is a total-body workout that can be done right from your chair, anywhere. It is perfect for office workers, travelers, and those with age-related movement limitations or special conditions. This book offers three programs. The *One-Hour Chair Program* is a full-body, low-impact workout that includes light aerobics and exercises to be done with or without weights. The *5-Day Short Program* features five compact workouts for those short on time. Finally, the *Ten-Minute Miracles* is a group of easy-to-do exercises perfect for anyone on the go.

160 pages ... 212 b/w photos ... Paperback ... $12.95 ... Hardcover $22.95

PEAK PERFORMANCE FITNESS: Maximizing Your Fitness Potential Without Injury or Strain

by Jennifer Rhodes, M.S.PT. Foreword by Joan E. Edelstein

Jennifer Rhodes looks at the body as an integrated system and offers a step-by-step plan for developing cardiovascular capacity, strength, and flexibility based on your body type and posture. She gives real-life success stories of how her approach has helped clients, while detailed photographs and anatomical drawings illustrate the exercises. If you are serious about long-term health and want to get to your best body ever, this book will help you redefine the way you exercise and move.

160 pages ... 46 b/w photos ... 31 illus. ... Paperback ... $14.95

ORDER FORM

NAME

ADDRESS

CITY/STATE   ZIP/POSTCODE

PHONE   COUNTRY (outside of U.S.)

TITLE	QTY	PRICE	TOTAL
Sudden Menopause (paperback)		@ $15.95	
Prices subject to change without notice			

Please list other titles below:

		@ $	
		@ $	
		@ $	
		@ $	
		@ $	
		@ $	
		@ $	
		@ $	

Check here to receive our book catalog ☐   free

Shipping Costs

First book: $3.00 by bookpost, $4.50 by UPS, Priority Mail, or to ship outside the U.S. Each additional book: $1.00
For rush orders and bulk shipments call us at (800) 266-5592

TOTAL	_____
Less discount @____%	(_____)
TOTAL COST OF BOOKS	_____
CA residents add 7½% sales tax	_____
Shipping & handling	_____
TOTAL ENCLOSED *Please pay in U.S. funds only*	========

☐ Check ☐ Money Order ☐ Visa ☐ MasterCard ☐ Discover

Card #_____ Exp. date_____

Signature_____

Complete and mail to:
Hunter House Inc., Publishers
PO Box 2914, Alameda CA 94501-0914
Website: www.hunterhouse.com
Orders: (800) 266-5592 or **email: ordering@hunterhouse.com**
Phone (510) 865-5282 Fax (510) 865-4295

SMP 06/2001